Second Edition

HUMAN
CARING
SCIENCE

A Theory of Nursing

JEAN WATSON, PhD, RN, AHN-BC, FAAN

Distinguished Professor of Nursing
Murchinson-Scoville Endowed Chair in Caring Science
University of Colorado, Denver
College of Nursing
Denver, Colorado

Founder: Watson Caring Science Institute
Boulder, Colorado

D1594545

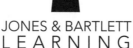

JONES & BARTLETT
LEARNING

World Headquarters

Jones & Bartlett Learning
40 Tall Pine Drive
Sudbury, MA 01776
978-443-5000
info@jblearning.com
www.jblearning.com

Jones & Bartlett Learning
Canada
6339 Ormindale Way
Mississauga, Ontario L5V 1J2
Canada

Jones & Bartlett Learning
International
Barb House, Barb Mews
London W6 7PA
United Kingdom

Jones & Bartlett's books and products are available through most bookstores and online booksellers. To contact Jones & Bartlett Learning directly, call 800-832-0034, fax 978-443-8000, or visit our website, www.jblearning.com.

Substantial discounts on bulk quantities of Jones & Bartlett Learning publications are available to corporations, professional associations, and other qualified organizations. For details and specific discount information, contact the special sales department at Jones & Bartlett Learning via the above contact information or send an email to specialsales@jblearning.com.

The author, editor, and publisher have made every effort to provide accurate information. However, they are not responsible for errors, omissions, or for any outcomes related to the use of the contents of this book and take no responsibility for the use of the products and procedures described. Treatments and side effects described in this book may not be applicable to all people; likewise, some people may require a dose or experience a side effect that is not described herein. Drugs and medical devices are discussed that may have limited availability controlled by the Food and Drug Administration (FDA) for use only in a research study or clinical trial. Research, clinical practice, and government regulations often change the accepted standard in this field. When consideration is being given to use of any drug in the clinical setting, the health care provider or reader is responsible for determining FDA status of the drug, reading the package insert, and reviewing prescribing information for the most up-to-date recommendations on dose, precautions, and contraindications, and determining the appropriate usage for the product. This is especially important in the case of drugs that are new or seldom used.

Production Credits
Publisher: Kevin Sullivan
Editorial Assistant: Rachel Shuster
Production Editor: Amanda Clerkin
Associate Marketing Manager: Katie Hennessy
V.P., Manufacturing and Inventory Control: Therese Connell
Composition: Paw Print Media
Cover Design: Kristin E. Parker
Cover Image: © Helen E. Grose/Dreamstime.com
Printing and Binding: Malloy, Inc.
Cover Printing: Malloy, Inc.

Library of Congress Cataloging-in-Publication Data
Watson, Jean, 1940–
  Human caring science : a theory of nursing / Jean Watson.—2nd ed.
    p. ; cm.
  Rev. ed. of: Nursing : human science and human care / Jean Watson. c1999.
  Includes bibliographical references and index.
  ISBN-13: 978-1-4496-2810-9 (alk. paper)
  ISBN-10: 1-4496-2810-9 (alk. paper)
  1. Nursing—Philosophy. 2. Caring. I. Watson, Jean, 1940– Nursing : human science and human care. II. Title.
  [DNLM: 1. Philosophy, Nursing. 2. Nursing Theory. WY 86]
  RT84.5.W367 2012
  610.73–dc22
                          2010048642

6048

Printed in the United States of America
15 14 13 12 11   10 9 8 7 6 5 4 3 2 1

Dedication

To all my relations.

Dedication

Contents

Preface

The aim of the revision to this book is to continue to resolve some pending conceptual and philosophical disciplinary problems about nursing and its evolution/maturity into the 21st century and beyond. It is my hope that this revision/rewrite also will guide others to join me in my quest to elucidate the human caring process in nursing, preserve humanity and the concept of the person/inner life world of the patient in our science/systems/society, and reintroduce love and healing into our educational and clinical practices.

I continue to share the timeless quote I saw in Bombay, India, during my first visit to that country; the quote was framed and hung on the bedroom wall of the children's room in a physician's home I was visiting. It read: "Life is not a problem to be solved, but a mystery to be lived." This saying expresses some of my own conceptual conflicts about nursing. Because the practice of nursing is in itself a mystery to be lived, some of nursing's foci and thus human living-dying experiences are not ones that necessarily can be solved. Nevertheless, how can I, or we, go about highlighting "the mystery to be lived" well enough to have it valued, esteemed, "seen," developed, and incorporated into nursing education, practice, and research?

In setting forth my ideas about nursing and people in general, I found that having distance helps clarify my thoughts. I wrote the original manuscript in Perth, Western Australia, some 4,000 miles from home, overlooking the calm, peaceful Swan River, feeling the fresh sea breeze from the Indian Ocean. Now to continue this journey for the second edition, I find myself in my sacred space in Mexico, Mar de Cortez, where I seek time out for my writing and reflecting in the midst of a too busy life. I also capture the writing in Boulder, Colorado, my home for over 30 years, as well as moments in transition with my work in the world today.

Here in Mexico I take time to be quiet, to be still in the midst of sea and sounds of nature, to create and write from an inner place guided by my personal/

professional experiences and longings for nursing and humankind at this time in our world. Human caring beginning with self and radiating outward to other, environment, community, nation, world, Planet Earth and the universe, to infinite mystery beyond.

The human caring process in nursing is, I believe, connected to universal human struggles and human tasks, combined with the tearing and wounding that can happen to a person or a race, a culture, or a civilization. This intensely human process of nursing can be a struggle for the professional nurse during a time of human and cultural transitions, from a world of materialism, scientism, technological, human, and environmental control, and domination, leading to global mistrust and corruption of human values and practices, This transition and evolution of human consciousness, and somewhat of a crisis in human caring, is now complicated by global distress from human caring to eco-caring and survival of humanity and Planet Earth as we have known it.

In my first book, *Nursing: The Philosophy and Science of Caring* (1979, Boston: Little, Brown, reprinted by University Press of Colorado) and the revised edition (2008, Boulder: University Press of Colorado), I had no inclination to refer to my ideas as a theory. That earlier work was my attempt to solve some conceptual and empirical problems about nursing, what comprises nursing, and how various components of nursing relate to and direct education, practice, and research. The original, *Nursing: The Philosophy and Science of Caring* (1979) was, in fact, a treatise on nursing.

When formulating my ideas, I began to structure a set of beliefs and concepts and to organize a body of knowledge and principles underlying human behavior in health and illness. Through this process came the 10 "carative" factors in nursing. Although my work was not a scientific theory per se, I was indeed theorizing about nursing and consequently going through the beginning stages of developing my own "theory" of nursing.

The revised (2008) book is an extension of my lifelong career in nursing and scholarship in caring science. My orientation for this work remains within a "phenomenological existential-spiritual" realm. The evolved work builds on the original influences of Hegel, Marcel, Whitehead, Kierkegaard, and East-West psychology and philosophy.

In the past decade I have been influenced with an even greater expanded world view, a greater cosmology, now increasingly converging between and among indigenous cultures worldwide and what French philosopher Emmanuel Levinas named as the "Ethic of Belonging," reminding us that before our separate being we all belong to the universal infinite field of cosmic love (Levinas, 1969). Levinas identified this larger universal ethic as first principle and starting point for science. Thus, human science/human caring is grounded in this larger universal cosmology, as ethical starting point.

Sally Gadow's work on existential advocacy was also a source of influence and inspiration in refining and validating my original ideas. The evolving work has continued to deepen through remarkable international travel and living experiences, which now include more than 12 times around the world of nursing groups. My journeys have included profound cultural–spiritual personal/professional experiences, journeys, and encounters in New Zealand, Australia, Indonesia, Malaysia, Taiwan, Thailand, India, Colombia, Peru, Brazil, Japan, Philippines, China, Mexico, and Egypt and certainly experiences and learnings throughout Europe, the United States, Canada, and beyond.

Although this work is primarily helpful for graduate students in nursing, it is well suited also to faculty members and to students of upper division baccalaureate programs. Hopefully, it also will touch a need in professional nurses who are struggling with the day-to-day world of human caring in nursing.

Finally, the retitling of the book from *Nursing: Human Science and Human Care* to *Human Caring Science: A Theory of Nursing* reflects my evolution of framing and naming caring science as the disciplinary foundation for the nursing profession. That is, once one places the human and caring and even concepts of love and healing into a model of science, we have to acknowledge we have a different model of science that emerges from disciplinary maturity. Thus, it is at the theoretical and disciplinary level that we make more explicit the ethical, philosophical, moral values, the world view, and lens one holds toward knowing/being/doing in relation to human caring and humanity, health-illness, healing, suffering, living, dying, and all the vicissitudes of life that nurses experience every day.

You will also note that the words "human care" in the original book have been changed to "human caring" or "caring" to again convey a deeper human-to-human involvement and connection one to another, which goes beyond the more concrete notion of what can be implied with the term *human care*. That is, one can offer human care without caring for or caring about the other person, limiting the authentic ethical relational caring processes contained within this theory and unitary views of person and universe.

I hope this work provides greater clarity about my perspective on and approach to nursing as a mature discipline and caring–healing, health profession. In addition, I hope this book helps to maintain and elevate the standard of the nursing profession and improve the welfare of people receiving and delivering nursing care. Finally, I hope the ideas contained in this volume stimulate additional theory development by reaching out and touching the human mind and heart, contributing to the evolution of human consciousness by offering nursing a disciplinary specific theoretical foundation for its continued evolution.

Jean Watson

Acknowledgments

Acknowledgments go to all the nursing doctoral students at the University of Colorado since the start of the program in 1978, along with all the colleagues, students, faculty, and practitioners all over the globe who have been touched by and have touched me with the philosophy and theory of human caring. And to those nurses around the world who continue to believe in nursing's "new" caring science.

I express my gratitude to all those now connected with the Watson Caring Science Institute (WCSI) and its programs, the International Association of Human Caring and the Caritas Coach Educational program, as well as other activities and programs associated with the WCSI (www.watsoncaringscience.org).

Finally, I treasure Jennifer and Julie and my five grandchildren, Demitri, Alma, Theo, Gabriel, and Joseph, whose spirit and deep love is ever with me.

CHAPTER 1

Introduction:
Context for Theory Development

"And the language of science cannot be freed from ambiguity, any more than poetry can;—in spite of its tidy look, the structure of science is no more exact, in any ultimate and final sense, than that of poetry."

—J. BRONOWSKI, THE IDENTITY OF MAN

This work represents the development of a nursing theory—not a hard scientific theory that is absolute, verifiable, quantifiable, and rigidly testable and that leads to facts, truths, and axiomatized statements—but, nevertheless, a theory. It is a theory because it helps me "to see" more broadly and clearly, and it may be useful in solving some conceptual and empirical problems in nursing and in human sciences generally.

These views are presented with the hope that they may help others "to see," to view phenomena in a new or different way, perhaps to develop or to attempt a new starting point, to use a new lens when focusing on the phenomena of human experiences in caring–healing, health, and illness. Ideas are proposed about how nursing connects with and serves people, which, in turn, advances society's knowledge of human conditions and advances nursing's contribution to the welfare of society, helping to sustain humanity and human caring in the world.

CLARIFYING THE MEANING OF THEORY

I love the notion of theory from the Latin word *Theoria*, which literally means "to see." More specifically, a theory can be thought of as an imaginative grouping of knowledge, ideas, and experience that are represented symbolically and seek to illuminate a given phenomenon. "Science," scientific development, and theory development are all related to art, the humanities, and philosophy. All are related to imagination, creativity, mystery, personal problem-solving, and attempts at "being" in relation to the universe. An artist is as scientific as a scientist is artistic. I reject methods that ascribe an increasing degree of reality to numbers and factual information, when at the same time the human need for meaning, aesthetics, wholeness, faith, inspiration, and a sense of wonder, mystery, and discovery is pushed farther into the background. Indeed, the definition of theory that continues to inspire me is *Theoria*, "to see." How can we do things differently if we cannot "see" what is right in front of us and have a conceptual lens for how to engage with our own phenomena?

Another important critical dimension to theory is to provide language, voice, and purpose to what is often invisible, such as caring and love, "old, unfamiliar words and actions, unnamed, not seen, because not looked for, but hidden in the stillness behind the scenes," to paraphrase T.S. Eliot.

I reject definitions and interpretations of science and scientific inquiry that bury the quest for discovery, beauty, creativity, and a higher sense of spirit, of being-in-the-world; acknowledging that we are all connected. In our own way we are relating to that which is greater than all, seeking harmony, right-order, and relation with the greater universe.

I want nursing to move beyond objectivism, verification, rigid operations, and definitions and concern itself more with meaning, relationships, intersubjective and intrasubjective context, and patterns; notions of evolving consciousness, intentionality, transpersonal, transcendent notions of caring and healing. I want nursing to be more concerned with the pursuit of hidden truths and new insights, developments of new knowledge in relation to human experiences in caring–healing, health and illness, and to make new discoveries of how to *be* in a professional human caring–healing relationship with individuals to better serve humankind and global civilization. As Lauden (1977, p. 81–82) states,

> Many of the theories within any evolving research tradition will be mutually inconsistent rivals, precisely because some theories represent attempts, within the framework of the traditions to improve and connect with their predecessors. A research tradition is a set of general assumptions about the entities and processes in a domain of study and about the appropriate methods to be used for investigating the problems and constructing the theories in the domain. A successful research tradition is one which leads, via its component theories, to the adequate solution of an ever increasing range of empirical and conceptual problems.

The broader task underlying this work is to help clarify the nature of nursing's contribution to humankind by way of an ethical, philosophical, and theoretical perspective that helps to solve some empirical and conceptual problems related to the disciplinary foundation that underlies nursing science and seeks the preservation of the whole person and human caring, which is humanity at the deepest level. Nursing's challenge of the day is to break the old bonds of preoccupation with procedures, facts per se, and rigid definitions of Era I science, evidence, strict rationalism, operationalism, variable manipulation, and metaphors of body as machine. We must recognize other ways of knowing and alternative, expanding/evolving views of science and changing world views and cosmology of the universe, and of reality itself, which are radiating around the world. This evolving consciousness/world view shift is uniting us globally to attend to human caring and eco-caring for health and survival of Planet Earth.

Further, it is critical for nursing at this turn in history, the centenary of Nightingale, to be clear about sustaining a meaningful ethical, philosophical foundation to its science and theories, lest we lose our way in this chaotic, post-post modern era of change, chaos, and confusion. Nurses now are invited to become visionary leaders of hope, helping self and others to envision and awaken to new possibilities, an expanding, evolving consciousness, and work to co-create, shape intentional transformative world view change, rather than conform to outdated modes that no longer work for nursing, medicine, patients, self, systems, society nor humanity.

Thus, now we come face to face with a global shift in the universe, an awakening of human consciousness, and a new reality, reminding us of our connection with all living things and the need to consider nursing in relation to a unitary world view of science and life itself. This shift is contained within a deeper "Ethic of Belonging" to this infinite universal field, as we are evolving as well as surviving as a civilization or a planet (Levinas, 1969; Watson, 2005, 2008). This deeper ethical starting point has been described as Caring Science as Sacred Science (Watson, 2005), acknowledging that we are all connected on this fragile Planet Earth and as nurses we work with the life force, the mystery, miracles within the human–environment–infinite field that contains all.

Nursing is now in a new place, allowing for diverse methodologies, modalities, and approaches to study through various forms of inquiry, practice, and research that do not exhaust the meaning of the so-called facts or findings; these new parameters range from empirical to transpersonal/transcendent/metaphysical. We continue to develop methods that retain the human context and allow for advancement of knowledge about the lived world of human experiences, deepening our understanding of human caring, healing, wholeness, and health and well-being.

My position at this point takes us beyond the original human science context to a caring science framework, which invites the evolving nature of humankind and provides a rich ethical, moral, and philosophical foundation for the theory of human caring and, perhaps more importantly, for the profession itself. It invites an expanding epistemology and allows multiple forms of knowing and knowledge sources, human caring science incorporating art, humanities and clinical sciences, along with underlying "Ethic of Belonging" as a starting point/world view/cosmology for nursing and human caring and healing. Thus, nursing as a human science/caring science cannot be considered qualitatively continuous with conventional, reductionistic, scientific epistemology, separatist ontology, and restrictive methodologies. However, this view of knowing and human caring science is large enough to accommodate all forms of knowledge, inviting an open world view, expanding epistemologies, diversity of methodologies, and new forms of caring praxis, consistent with complexity and evolution of humanity and any health illness phenomena and healing experiences.

CONCEPTS

Because concepts are the basic building blocks for any theory, it is helpful to examine different ways in which concepts are treated by a theorist as a starting point for theory development.

Concepts and definitional terms in a given theory may extend on a horizontal continuum from the very absolute or concrete to the very relative or abstract (Figure 1-1). A theorist's starting point on the concrete–abstract continuum influences further directions for the theory. Any theory's structure, flexibility, utility, and so on are influenced by how the basic concepts are treated in the beginning stages; all other aspects of the work flow from that starting point.

Let's take a concept as elusive as nursing and even caring. The way the concept is treated may range from a very absolute, specific, concrete set of actions, tasks, and behaviors that one can directly observe and measure to extend to the very abstract, dynamic, philosophical ideal of nursing that is relativistic and placed within the unitary transformative context (or simultaneity paradigm). This perspective suggests a constantly changing, unitary dynamic process with different meanings and a different world view, including personal meaning, evolution of human consciousness, setting one's intentionality, and, thus, changing views of our very reality.

This continuum can be reframed in contemporary nursing literature as ranging from particulate–deterministic foci toward interactive–relational foci all the way to simultaneity/unitary–transformative cosmology/world view. Each conceptual starting point and location with respect to theoretical orientation points us toward different theories that can help to solve conceptual–empirical–ethical–theoretical issues. Furthermore, nursing and its image, world view, metaphors, and concept

---

Figure 1-1   Horizontal concept continuum.

Concrete	Abstract
Measurable	Theoretical
Observable	Ideals

may be codefined by the patient/family, community, society, and evolved humanity itself.

If a concept were placed somewhere in the middle of the concrete–abstract continuum, it may suggest a balanced view of the concept under question. In other words, the concept of nursing (and caring) may be treated in such a way that abstractions are allowed for, but abstract notions represent empirical reality to a degree that is comprehensible by others, both in philosophic, intellectual terms and in the world of practice.

If the concept of nursing is placed in the middle of the continuum, for example, nursing may be defined in such a way that it incorporates the action, doing, behavioral aspects of nursing but also allows for some relativistic notions such as the meaning that nursing may have to the experiencing patient. It may allow for the nursing (caring) presence to exist in a patient's mind, even if the nurse is not present physically. Such a balanced development of the concept of nursing provides both for objective and subjective dimensions of nursing with some specific measurable, observable aspects but also for some abstract, theoretical aspects that may or may not be measurable in behavioral terms but may be understandable and meaningful from a patient's experience and helpful conceptually within a theory.

In addition to the absolute–relative continuum as a starting point, another continuum can be vertically superimposed. This can be referred to as a vertical static–dynamic continuum (Figure 1-2). For example, could the way in which a concept is defined result in some external laws, universal truths, and certainties? If so, that may be useful, but there is also the danger that the definition may become static and deadened after verification. On the other hand, if the concept is viewed as dynamic, temporal, changing, and unfinished, the expression of the concept may allow for diversity, lack of certainty, paradox, and evolution, opening it to creative emergence and envisioning infinite possibilities.

These starting points on how the beginning concepts of any theory are expressed and defined determine where the theory ends up and to what extent it is useful in describing, explaining, understanding, and "seeing" the phenomena in question. Furthermore, the starting point on the concrete–abstract and static–dynamic continua also determines what methodologies are suitable for further scientific work, theory development, and research.

If the starting point for concept expression is at the concrete end of the horizontal continuum and the static point on the vertical continuum, then the scientific perspective of the theory is one of verification, absolutes, and measurables, including acceptance of truths, laws, and facts once they are tested. If a concept is placed on the abstract–dynamic ends of the two continua, then the scientific perspective is consistent with a view of science as discovery rather

Figure 1-2   Horizontal and vertical concept continua. (Vertical continuum idea attributed to Dr. Glenn Webster.)

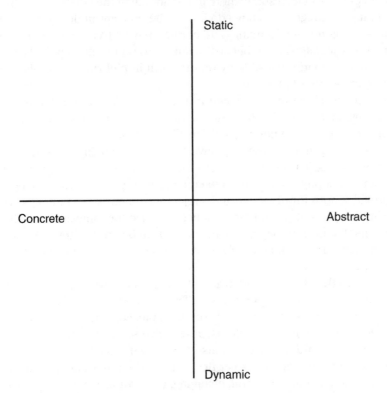

than verification, a pursuit of meaning and understanding that may be less than true but may hold promise for new ways of knowing, seeing, or answering questions, albeit tentative.

The verification–acceptance method of science is more concerned with science as a finished product. The discovery–pursuit method of science is more concerned with science as a process that is continuous, ongoing, and unfinished. To allow for movement of a concept on the vertical–horizontal axis, it is more useful to avoid being locked into either end of the two continua. However, depending on one's approach to science (as a product to be verified and accepted or as a process to be discovered and pursued), a theorist may end up on different points on the two continua. The theorist's orientation toward science influences his or her starting point for developing and defining the specific concepts that become the foundation and building blocks of the theory. In turn, the starting point for developing the concepts determines the methodologies and approaches to theory development, theory structure, and theory use. Thus, the starting point determines the end. The clearer one is about the starting point, the more one can see where or why one may end up in a certain place. One can also begin to recognize why a given theory's use was limited if the method for further work was inconsistent with the starting point. Some theories, for example, are investigated by verification methods related to science as a product when the theoretical concepts are more consistent with process discovery, pursuant to methods related to science as process. When that happens, the theory often dies. This has frequently occurred in periods of nursing theory developments.

There has been intellectual confusion in nursing as to which continua should operate; there have been some conceptual inconsistencies between and among some of the dimensions. Often, there are indications that concepts should be open, fluid, changing, and consistent with complexity, relationships, and context of human behavior and nursing science, but ideas have frequently been trapped by applications of rigid testability and methods of verification and acceptance that are not consistent with nursing as an evolving human caring science. There also has been some bootlegging of nursing concepts into molds of other disciplines that are not adequate for nursing as human caring science. At the same time, nursing, over the past few decades, has recognized that it can broaden its perspective on science, consistent with the changing nature of the history and philosophy of science, and explore numerous methods for advancing knowledge. There is a reawakening of consciousness and confidence for nursing to pursue nursing/caring science consistent with its own heritage and tradition that is related to the deeply human dimensions of science, to nursing, and to human caring–healing relational, contextual, even metaphysical phenomena and practices. For example, as a reminder, as soon as one places the human and phenomenon of human caring and concepts such a healing, wholeness, and even Love into a model of science, one has an entirely new view and different view of science. It requires an ethical and relational, contextual, evolving world view and starting point in that the human can never be "set" and localized in time and space and exists beyond the body's physical realm.

Before proceeding I would like to place my own theoretical perspective on the continua so the reader knows my starting point (Figure 1-3). Consistent with my views of science, specifically human caring science, I am concerned with process, the method of discovery, and the pursuit of hidden meanings, often mysterious, spirit-filled unknowns in nature living, dying, and the evolving universe; the sacred circle of life itself. Therefore, I place my ideas toward the far right-hand side of the abstract end of the horizontal continuum and toward the lower end of the vertical axis, associated with dynamic movement and lack of

Figure 1-3   Concept continua—concrete to abstract and static to dynamic.

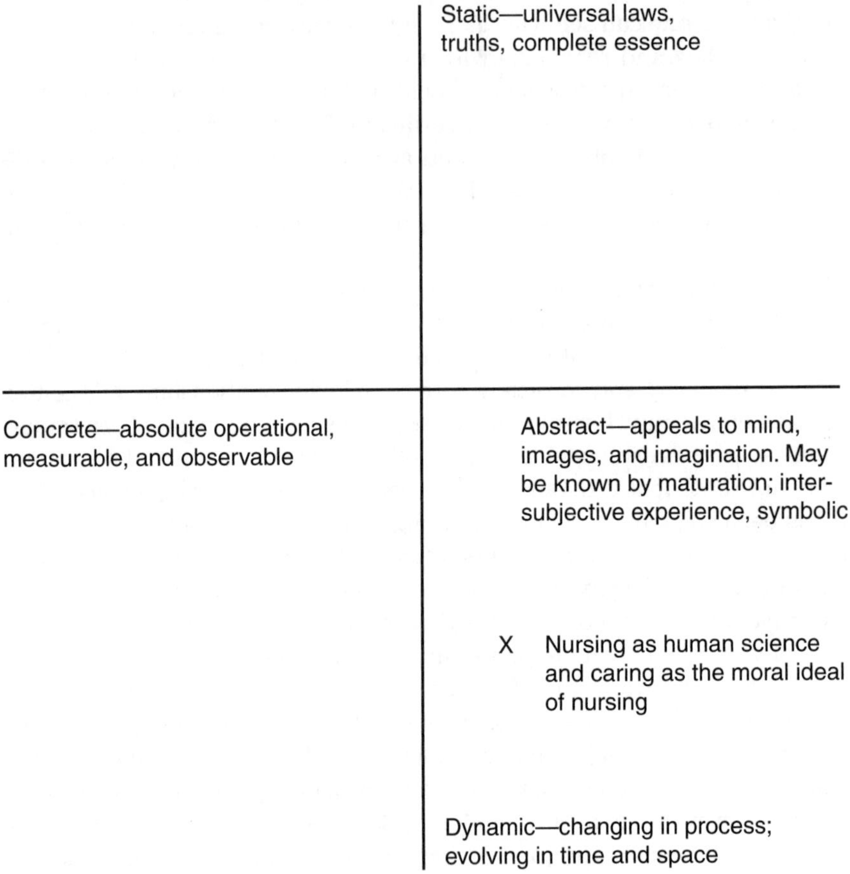

Static—universal laws, truths, complete essence

Concrete—absolute operational, measurable, and observable

Abstract—appeals to mind, images, and imagination. May be known by maturation; inter-subjective experience, symbolic

X   Nursing as human science and caring as the moral ideal of nursing

Dynamic—changing in process; evolving in time and space

certainties. At the same time, however, I am interested in movement back and forth and up and down on the dimensions—but my starting point is more toward the lower, right quadrant.

Any phase of theory development, such as concept definitions, concept representation, formulation of propositions, checks with empirical world for meaning, or clarification, may be more or less concrete–abstract or static–dynamic, depending on the theory and the theorist's world view and research tradition. For example, one can ask the following questions:

- Do the concepts in the theory induce a mental representation or high level abstraction? A behavioral inner mental/imaginative representation or a physical representation?
- Is the concept dynamic or time dependent or capable of transcending time, space, and physicality?
- Is the focus micro or macro?
- Is the scope partial or comprehensive?
- Is the outcome more descriptive where abstractions are visualized, metaphorical, and imagined or reduced to concrete language and words and/or numbers that are devoid of fuller meanings?
- Is the outcome restricted to only the operationalized definitions and observable events or open to continual theorizing, evolving?

Figure 1-4   Placement of Roy's and Rogers' theory of concept continua.

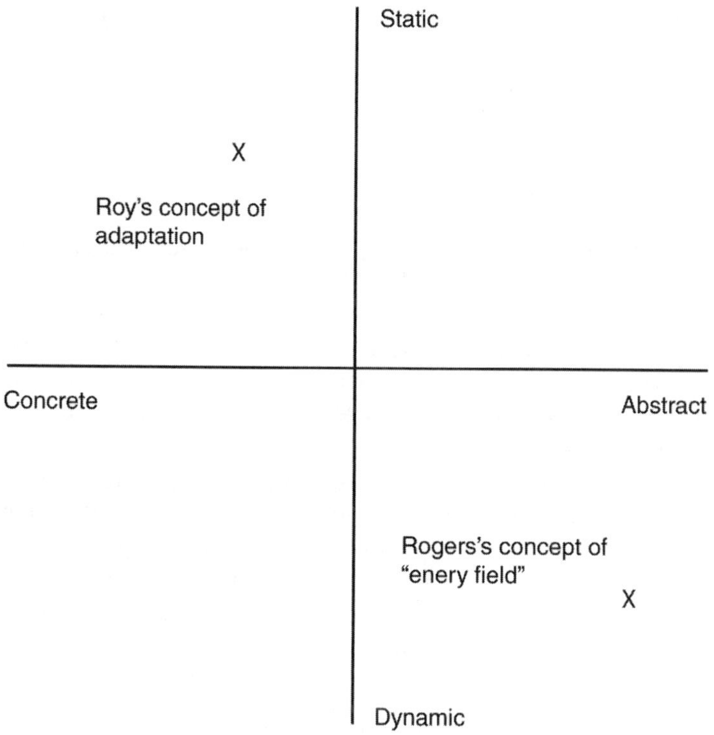

Static

X
Roy's concept of
adaptation

Concrete   Abstract

Rogers's concept of
"enery field"
                                                    X

Dynamic

- Is the focus on what ought to be (moral idealism/moral imperatives) or what is (practical realism)?
- Is there a high level of generalization at one level but a lack of specific facts and details at a more concrete, individual level (Figure 1-4)?

Consider the following illustrations and examples from nursing theory: Martha Rogers' (1970, 1994) theory of nursing and concept of energy field and Roy's (1976) concept of adaption. Rogers' concept of energy field is defined as electrical in nature in a continual state of flux and varies continuously in its intensity, density, and extent. The concept is broad, abstract, theoretical, and even metaphysical (beyond physical); it has a great deal of generalization but is void of specific facts. It helps one to see, comprehend, and grasp an essence without spelling out details of specific behavior; it evokes higher level mental images.

Roy's (1976) original concept of adaptation includes three classes of stimuli: (1) focal stimuli, (2) contextual stimuli, and (3) residual stimuli. As such, adaptation results from a response to a stimulus. This concept is placed in the concrete–static one because there is a limited generalization to higher levels of mental images. The concept is limited to specific stimuli that are more detailed and factual, measurable entities but is void of high-level generalization. It may help one to see immediate presenting behavior but does not help in grasping an essence or a higher abstract mental image, because it is concerned more with specific observable behavior of a given time. This perspective is useful for assessing and guiding one's thinking and actions for very practical presenting phenomena at a concrete, more biological level.

These two examples illustrate a macro (comprehensive) perspective (Rogers') and a more micro (partial) perspective (Roy's). Sometimes, different dictates and orientations have been dismissed under the guise of a science–nonscience schism. Consequently, a perspective that is too global and too abstract, even if it is rich and powerful as a mental device, is sometimes discredited. Likewise, depending on one's approach to science (whether the concern is with verification and product rather than discovery and process), one's preference is for one theory or the other. What is perhaps more useful in science, and certainly nursing, is this: (1) to be clear about one's particular leanings, (2) to encourage a diversity of approaches for theory development in nursing, and (3) to select an approach consistent with one's own values and beliefs. Preferable also is a theory that allows placement on the specificity–generalization scale and the concrete–abstract and static–dynamic continua that is consistent with the nature of nursing phenomena in question within the theory.

NEW LENS FOR SEEING NURSING

Nurse scientists and practitioners must treasure some of their nonlineari-ties and other unexpected results and avoid preconceptions based on ingrained ideas. We in nursing are moving away from homogeneity of thinking and seeking new breakthroughs and developing new ways of seeing the usual. Maybe at some level, like psychology, nursing is metaparadigmatic. Thus, theories may need some isolation to evolve to prevent their dilution and submersion into the common and ordinary.

Nursing/caring science as a focus has to work at changing its lens to see anew and appreciate some of its beauty, art, and humanity as well as its empir-ical clinical science. Perhaps the issue for nursing is to acknowledge again that once the human and caring are involved, it is not like the traditional sciences—it requires its own lens, orientation, ethic, and starting point for its descriptions; it possesses its own phenomena and needs its own range of diverse methods for clarification of its own concepts and their meanings, relationships, and context; its own expanded forms of inquiry, which can range from hard science clinical investigations at the biological level all the way to philosophical–ethical inquiry to the latest turn in reflective practice narratives, interpretative forms of inquiry, including performance and aesthetic installations and so on.

Such a range of forms of inquiry attest to the notion of causality, which cannot be carried over from the natural sciences to nursing and human caring knowledge and practices. The human-to-human caring relationships are mutual and life-giving and life-receiving for both nurses and others and cannot be explained or understood with a positivistic, deterministic, materialistic mind set.

When one looks back over the history of nursing science, it has not had one sure sense of direction but several quite unsure directions and various research traditions. I sometimes refer to this past struggle as nursing having "ontological insecurity," that is, nursing has been unclear about its own standing in that the pressures from objective views of science, methodological dictates, medical preoccupation, and clinical physical foci and restrictions have often taken nursing off course from its own development and clarity.

The apparent differences between nursing and other branches of science may result from the difficulty of the context, processes, and concepts involved, such as nursing, caring, humans, life, human relationships, health, healing, dying, and so on. These are not just clinical, empirical, and biophysical phenomena, these are also ethical, philosophical, spiritual, and even metaphysical phenomena that have to be named and honored as major unique phenomenon of nursing and caring science. From Nightingale onward, nursing continues to embrace a deep ethical, philosophical, and moral orientation toward humanity itself and toward its covenant with society to sustain human caring, human dignity, wholeness, and health care in home/community as well as clinical settings/hospitals. Thus, this orientation and deep commitment to humanity and caring phenomena have not always been understood by the outer world of medicine and conventional science.

> *"Our educational and epistemological and ethical models have to rise to the twenty-first-century occasion as a moral invitation and responsibility to create new or at least different educational and pedagogical options for science and society alike."*
>
> —WATSON (2008, P. 256)

It is significant that many of the problems of nursing/caring science, theory, and research are now being explored more systematically. A variety of efforts is being pursued to bring a selected body of knowledge into a disciplinary framework for studying, researching, educating, and practicing nursing (see, for example, Newman et al., 1991; Boykin & Schoenhofer, 2001; Watson & Smith, 2002; Benner et al., 2010; Hills & Watson, 2011; Smith & McCarthy, 2010; Watson, 2005, 2008).

REDEFINING SCIENCE

The dominant features of conventional science and medicine that make it anomalous to nursing and human caring science have been stated in different ways but can be summed up in three characteristics—objectivism, scientism, and technism. These are shared by the two most influential philosophical systems in the history of science, Cartesianism and positivism.

Nursing continues to undergo a questioning and lack of clarity as to whether it should continue to align itself with conventional 'evidence-based' science to improve practice or to extend science in favor of some other approach to reality. It is inappropriate and irresponsible to discard extant views of science and discount scientific progress, but at the same time science as traditionally viewed and presented must be questioned and challenged in nursing and human caring sciences.

As soon as we are explicit about a unitary world view and about the unity of a human, caring, environmental, nature universe in a model of science, we have ushered in a different model of science. In that caring, human, environmental, nature universe is a unified field, and patterns upon patterns of reality exist within the larger unitary, cosmological world view held by Nightingale and Rogers and now by other contemporary nursing theorists such as Parse, Newman, and Watson.

We are at a stage in human evolution not only of acknowledging the revisioning of science but also of acknowledging an evolving and changing world view of the universe in which we reside; moving from human caring to eco-caring if the planet Earth and humans are to survive into this century and this millennium. Thus, now we humbly admit a moral and ethical starting point, honoring the wholeness of being in the world and unitary view of human-caring-environment and the larger universe. As such, the world view of science is relational and relativistic and not an absolute separatist view of reality and phenomena.

It is appropriate that nurses continue to ethically critique and question the impersonal, objective model of the human in science, adhering to the personal unique, often indescribable human caring–healing relational gestalt experiences. The human caring science paradigm for nursing must allow human phenomena to emerge and still be investigated; however, the method must be such that the dynamics of relationship and unknowns are allowed, explored, and honored.

Without wanting to create an additional set of false dichotomies between science and art or between traditional–medical–natural science models and human caring science and nursing models, Table 1-1 sets forth some of the major differences/dialectics that help clarify nursing's scientific context.

Table 1-1 is not intended to reinforce differences but acknowledge the dance of dialectics between and among these dynamics, or to heighten awareness of different assumptions. These differences/dialectics direct our thinking and behavior and need to be examined continually. Sometimes, the differences can be reconciled through a dialectical process of thesis, antithesis, and synthesis. Some remain as differences and need to be at least acknowledged because they represent different starting points and lead us in different directions.

As a way of summarizing my ideas within a context of theory development, Chapter 9 provides a synopsis and a structural overview of my theory of human caring. It also offers the reader a succinct analysis of the theory and its major components, including subject matter, values, goals, agents of change, caring-healing modalities and nursing therapeutics, perspective, context, approach, and method.

Table 1-1 Differing Perspectives Between Traditional Science and Human Caring Science

Traditional Medical Natural Science Context	Emerging Alternative Nursing Human Caring Science
Normative	Ipsative
Reductionistic	Transactional/transpersonal/transcendent
Mechanistic	Metaphysical/spirit filled Humanistic—contextual/evolving
Method centered	Phenomena centered
Neutrality of values	Value laden; values acknowledged, clarified
Disease centered on pathology–physiology	Subjective inner whole person: meaning Human inner subjective response meanings of human condition
Ethics of "science"	Unitary Ethic of Belonging/oneness/ connectedness
More quantitative	More qualitative/combination allowing all forms of knowledge; diverse forms of inquiry
Absolutes, givens, laws	Relativism, dynamic unfolding; creative emergence
Human as object	Human as subject
Objective experiences	Subjective–intersubjective experiences
Facts	Experience, meaning

REFERENCES

Benner, P., Sutphen, M., Leonard, V., & Day, L. (2010). *Educating nurses: A call for radical transformation. The Carnegie Report for the Advancement of Teaching.* San Francisco: Jossey-Bass.

Boykin, A., & Schoenhofer, S. (2001). *Nursing as caring.* Sudbury, MA: Jones and Bartlett.

Hills, M., & Watson, J. (2011). *Creating a caring science curriculum. Emancipatory pedagogies for nursing education.* New York: Springer.

Lauden, L. (1977). *Progress and its problems: Toward a theory of scientific growth* (pp. 81–82). Berkeley, CA: University of California Press.

Levinas, E. (1969). *Totality and infinity.* Pittsburgh, PA: Duquesne University. [14th printing, 2000.]

Newman, M., Sime, A. M., Corcoran-Perry, S. A. (1991). The focus of the discipline of nursing. *Advances in Nursing Science. 13*, 1–14.

Rogers, M. (1970). *An introduction to the theoretical basis of nursing* (pp. 90, 91, 92, 104, 113). Philadelphia: F.A. Davis.

Rogers, M. (1994). The science of unitary human beings. *Nursing Science Quarterly, 2,* 33–35.

Roy, Sister C. (1976). *Introduction to nursing: An adaption model* (pp. 22, 30–32, 38). Englewood Cliffs, NJ: Prentice-Hall.

Smith, M., & McCarthy, P. (2010). Disciplinary knowledge in nursing education: Going beyond the blueprints. *Nursing Outlook, 58,* 44–51.

Watson, J. Smith, M. C. (2002). Caring science and science of unitary human being: A transtheoretical discourse for nursing knowledge development. *Journal Advanced Nursing, 37*(5), 452–461.

Watson, J. (2005). *Caring science as sacred science.* Philadelphia: F.A. Davis.

Watson, J. (2008). *Nursing. The philosophy and science of caring.* Boulder, CO: University Press of Colorado.

BIBLIOGRAPHY

Abdellah, F. G. (1969). The nature of nursing science. *Nursing Research, 18,* 390.

Alexandersson, C. (1981). Amedeo Giorgi's empirical phenomenology (publication no. 3). Swedish Council for Research in Humanities and Social Sciences, Department of Education, University of Goteborg, Sweden.

Dennis, N. (1982). New methods for research. Paper presented at Western Australian Institute of Technology, Western Australia, May.

Flaskerud, J. H., & Halloran, E. (1980). Areas of agreement in nursing theory development. *Advances in Nursing Science, 3*(1).

Gaylin, W. (1976). *Caring.* New York: Knopf.

Giorgi, A. (1970). *Psychology as a human science.* New York: Harper & Row.

Hall, L. E. (1964). Nursing—What is it? *Canadian Nurse, 60,* 150–154.

Henderson, V. (1964). The nature of nursing. *American Journal of Nursing, 64,* 62–68.

Hyde, A. (1975–1977). *The phenomenon of caring: Part I–Part IV* (vols. 10–12). American Nursing Foundation.

Johnson, D. (1978). State of art of theory development in nursing. In National League for Nursing (Ed.), *Theory development: What, why, and how.* New York: National League for Nursing.

Johnson, R. (1975). *In quest of a new psychology.* New York: Human Sciences Press.

King, I. (1971). *Toward a theory for nursing.* New York: Wiley.

Koch, S. (Ed.). (1959). *Psychology: A study of science.* New York: McGraw-Hill.

Koch, S. (1969). Psychology cannot be a coherent science. *Psychology Today, 3*(4), 64, 66.

Kohler, W. (1947). *Gestalt psychology.* New York: Liveright.

Kreuter, F. R. (1957). What is good nursing care? *Nursing Outlook, 5,* 302–305.

Lauden, L. (1977). *Progress and its problems: Toward a theory of scientific growth.* Berkeley, CA: University of California Press.

Leininger, M. (1969). Conference on the nature of science in nursing. Introduction: Nature of science in nursing. *Nursing Research, 18*(5).

Leininger, M. (1979). Foreword. In J. Watson (Ed.). *Nursing: The philosophy and science of caring*. Boston: Little, Brown.

Leininger, M. (Ed.). (1981). *Caring*. Thorofare, NJ: Charles B. Slack.

Levin, M. (1971). Holistic nursing. *Nursing Clinics of North America, 6*(2).

Marton, F. (1978). *Describing conceptions of the world around us. Reports from Institute of Education*. Goteborg, Sweden: University of Goteborg.

Marton, F., & Svensson, L. (1979). Conceptions of research in student learning. *Higher Education, 8.*

Mayerhoff, M. (1971). *On caring*. New York: Harper & Row.

Murphy, J. (Ed.). (1971). *Theoretical issues in professional nursing*. New York: Appleton-Century-Crofts.

Newman, M. (1979). *Theory development in nursing*. Philadelphia: F. A. Davis.

Nightingale, F. (1860). *Notes on nursing: What it is and what it is not*. New York: Appleton.

Norris, C. M. (Ed.). (1969). *Proceedings, First Nursing Theory Conference*. Kansas City, KS: University of Kansas Press, 1969.

Oiler, C. (1982). The phenomenological approach in nursing research. *Nursing Research, 31*(3), 178–181.

Omery, A. (1982). Phenomenology: A method for nursing research. *Advances in Nursing Science, 5*(2), 49–63.

Parse, R. R. (1981). *Man—Living health: A theory of nursing*. New York: Wiley.

Paterson, J. D., & Zderak, L. Y. (1976). *Humanistic nursing*. New York: Wiley.

Peplau, H. (1952). *Interpersonal relations in nursing*. New York: Putnam.

Pickering, M. (1980). Introduction to qualitative research methodology. Paper presented at the American Speech–Language and Hearing Association, Detroit, November.

Rist, R. C. (1977). On the relations among educational research paradigms: From disdain to detente. *Anthropology and Educational Quarterly, 8*, 42–49.

Rogers, M. (1970). *Theoretical basis of nursing*. Philadelphia: F. A. Davis.

Roy, Sister C. (1976). *Introduction to nursing: An adaptation model*. Englewood Cliffs, NJ: Prentice-Hall.

Stevens, B. (1979). *Nursing theory*. Boston: Little, Brown.

Spicker, S., & Gadow, S. (Eds.). (1980). *Nursing images and ideals*. New York: Springer.

Valle, R., & King, M. (1978). *Existential phenomenological alternatives for psychology*. New York: Oxford University Press.

Van Kaam, A. L. (1959). Phenomenological analysis: Exemplified by a study of the experience of being really understood. *Individual Psychology, 15*, 66–72.

Watson J. (1979). *Nursing: The philosophy and science of caring*. Boston: Little, Brown.

Watson, J. (1981a). Nursing's scientific quest. *Nursing Outlook, 29*(7), 413–416.

Watson, J. (1981b). Professional identity crisis—Is nursing finally growing up? *American Journal of Nursing, 81*, 1488–1490.

Watson, J. (1984). Reflections of new methodologies for study of human care. In M. Leininger (Ed.), *Qualitative methodologies in nursing*. New York: Grune & Stratton.

Yura, K., & Torres, G. (1975). *Today's conceptual frameworks within baccalaureate nursing programs* (17–25). National League for Nursing publication no. 15-1558. New York: National League for Nursing.

CHAPTER 2

Nursing as Human Caring Science

"To effectively interpret the truly great role that has been assigned her (sic), neither a liberal education nor a high degree of technical skill will suffice. The nurse must also be master of two tongues, the tongue of science and that of the people."

—Annie Warburton Goodrich (1973)

In some of my earlier writings I tried to present a case for nursing as an art and a science, making it more akin to a human science tradition and what I call the science of caring. A second position I have taken is that nursing has submerged both its scientific and artistic heritage in its scientific quest and more recent preoccupation with "evidence"-based practice (Watson, 2008). Such a position about the nature of nursing and nursing science is hardly unique. In fact, an exploration of the early writings on nursing shows similar ideas about the nature of nursing (Watson, 1981).

Even though nursing is still evolving and has yet to actualize the ideas and ideals of the early nursing leaders, including the Nightingale model of nursing, the most contemporary theories of nursing generally promote converging ideas about nursing, that is, they deal with expanding unitary, ethical, philosophical views of person-nature-environment-universe; expanding, evolving human consciousness; and life-sustaining caring–healing knowledge, patterns, and processes. As nursing progresses, it is breaking away from the traditional medical–scientific bondage and tending to develop its own scientific heritage. For example, contemporary themes of nursing converge across extant nursing theory: relativism, process, paradox, pattern, energy, consciousness, relationship, meaning, inner subjectivity, integral views of knowledge, intentionality, unitary views of reality, human-environment field, unitary person, wholeness, unity of mind-body-spirit, sacred nature of life force, spirit (Watson, 2005, 2008, 2011). The irony, paradoxically, is that although nursing and contemporary theories of nursing are converging, offering clarity and consistency and even maturity to nursing's caring science context and disciplinary foundation, the most current trend in nursing education and research is to disregard nursing theory and ignore nursing's disciplinary foundation, focusing more on conventional forms of evidence, methods, medical-institutional requirements, and procedures, thereby conforming to practices from the outer world of control, institutional pressures, and demands.

These converging and continuously emerging and evolving themes relate to nursing phenomena that go beyond and contain, but transcend, the bio-physical, material plane of existence and world view of separation (Watson, 2005, 2008, 2011). Witness all the work in nursing theory and evolution of the discourse in nursing as a discipline over the past two decades and more: shift toward critique of nature of nursing phenomena, nature of knowledge (episte-mology), critique of ontology (world view: what does it mean to be in the world?), critique of methodology (method should fit the phenomenon not forcing method onto phenomenon), and uncovering nursing and human caring–healing health phenomena as basis for disciplinary foundation of mature nursing (Newman, 1979, Newman et al., 1991; Boykin & Schoenhofer, 2001; Watson & Smith, 2002; Benner et al., 2010; Hills & Watson, 2011; Smith & McCarthy, 2010; Watson, 1999, 2005, 2008).

It appears that early nursing leaders as well as contemporary nursing theo-rists attempted to create a research tradition providing clarity and maturity of nursing's paradigm, moving from pre-paradigmatic to a mature paradigm status. This evolved clarity and maturity of nursing' disciplinary paradigm is what I framed as caring science—as the ethical, philosophical, and moral disciplinary foundation for a consistent, historical, and contemporary value-centered 21st century nursing (Watson, 2005, 2008; Hills & Watson, 2011).

In other words, all this momentum is to establish a set of general assumptions about the values, the ethical-philosophical context, the world view, the nature of knowledge, the entities and processes in the domain of study, and the appro-priate methods, transformative practices, policies, and leadership capacities to be used for investigating problems and generating and constructing theories guided by knowledge of phenomena of relevance to nursing (i.e., human-caring-healing-health phenomena), sacred life force and inner human subjective expe-riences, meaning of conditions and life situations, along with the relationship between and among the deep dimensions of an evolved humanity, of an evolved consciousness, toward a unitary world view (Watson, 1981, 1999, 2005, 2008).

Florence Nightingale, for example, talked of a "new art and a new science" and presented nursing as an act that required organized and scientific training (Nightingale, 1860). She did not create a false dichotomy between science and art. Her famous words follow (p. 355):

> Nursing is an art; and if it is to be made an art, it requires as exclusive a devotion, as hard a preparation as any painter's or sculptor's work.

Other views of nursing from Nightingale encompass the incredible use of facts and statistics in informing others of health problems:

All sciences of observation depend upon statistical methods—without these, [they] are blind empiricism. Make your facts comparable before deducing causes. . . . Insufficient number of observations; this is what one sees. (Nightingale, in Dossey, 2007:230).

Later, leaders such as Virginia Henderson, Lydia Hall, and Frances Krueter promoted concepts of nursing that were consistent with Nightingale's. Henderson, for example, defined the nurse's role as very subjective and qualitative. She believed the nurse should. . . get inside the skin of each of (her) patients in order to know what (he/she) needs (Henderson, 1964).

Likewise, Annie Goodrich, in paraphrasing the American nurse pioneer who had personal contact with Nightingale, nursing imbues the simplest acts with importance and instills a desire for the utmost skill and accuracy in performance. It commands devoted service, . . . a broad perspective, . . . rigorous analyses, close association with scientific findings, fine perceptions, (and) enduring tolerance born of understanding (Goodrich, 1973). I adopt the following common and broad themes from nursing's heritage about the nature of nursing:

1. A unitary view of the human as a unique, valued, and precious person in and of him- or herself to be cared for, respected, nurtured, understood, and assisted; in general, a philosophical view of a person as a whole person, honoring the unity of mind-body-spirit, continuous with the larger environmental field, the Planet Earth, and the cosmos infinite field of life itself. My work makes explicit the concept of soul by acknowledging the sacredness of life force, the human soul. Again, Nightingale indicated the care of the body can never be separate from care of the soul. This view of humanity honors the fact that we each belong and relate to the broader infinite field of life itself: the great mystery, the void, the source of life, the energy-spirit-consciousness-cosmic love, which is greater than any person. Thus, the human being cannot be defined as the sum of the parts but as a unified whole, whereby there is a oneness of all and everything is related to everything else.

2. An emphasis on the human inner subjective life world, the inner meaning of their existence, and the caring relationship and transaction between persons and their environment and how that affects health and healing in a broad sense.

3. An emphasis on the deeply human-to-human caring relationship and the caring moments between and among the nurse and other(s), acknowledging that the caring moment and the caring relationship affects the outcomes of health and healing.

4. An emphasis on the nonmedical processes of human caring and the nurse's caring relationship with persons, family, and community with various health–illness inner meaning and healing experiences.

5. A concern for health and healing that goes beyond any medical condition or treatment to help the other find their own best meaning, inner solutions, and self-guided pattern for health, healing, quality of living, transitioning, or dying.

6. A position that nursing knowledge and practice of human caring–healing is distinct from, but complementary to, medical knowledge and practice.

7. A concern with sustaining human dignity, preserving humanity, and facilitating self-knowing, self-control, self-caring, and even self-healing potential.

The problem today seems to be that nursing has yet to fully develop the *science and practices* of nursing in accordance with its *theories and its historic and contemporary mature disciplinary foundation.* Furthermore, conflicting paradigms operate among different views of nursing theory, nursing practice, and nursing research. This conflict is related to the fact that the early views of nursing that have persisted over time have still not been fully realized in education or in practice. The intervening years between the early leaders and contemporary theorists have been fraught with nursing's struggle to advance as a discipline and a profession. We have been caught between the paradigm of medical science with a body-part machine view of a person and the paradigm of natural, hard science with an emphasis on unsurpassable control, rigor, objectivism, neutrality of value, facts, procedures, skills, technology, and so on.

Consequently, in spite of its historical struggles, nursing nevertheless has come a long way. However, it is still evolving toward clarity of a meaningful philosophical foundation for its theories, its knowledge, and its science that is consistent with past, present, and future visions, images, and ideals of nursing leaders.

My position is a human science/caring science framework that provides a firm foundation for this next evolution of nursing as a distinct discipline and profession. This ancient and noble profession, which is over a hundred years old, must now converge with a global world view shift toward unity of all: our shared humanity, human-environment-Earth, and the larger cosmos.

HUMAN CARING SCIENCE

The notion of a "human science" was a term used by Giorgi (1970a) in his attempt to describe psychology as a discipline committed to the study of the person as a whole as opposed to the psychoanalytic or behaviorist views of psychology. This dilemma also applies to nursing's historical and traditional ties to medical science and to the psychoanalytic and behaviorist views of the person. This approach has been compounded with the continuing imprint of natural science, reductionist research methods, and current mindsets that perpetuate the hierarchy of empirical forms of evidence and outdated notions of what counts as a legitimate science. This dissonance lingers, in spite of major changes in theories, methodologies, and practices. The paradox is that nursing continues to adhere to its strong commitment to care of the whole person and a concern for the health-wholeness-healing of individuals and families and groups and communities.

As nursing has matured, it continued to critique the dissonance between and among its gold standard for science, what counts as knowledge and evidence, and the nature of human caring phenomena. Thus, focus on human science and caring science has surfaced in a variety of ways. To note views of Emmanuel Levinas (1969), ethics is the first principle for science and an "Ethic of Belonging" (to infinite cosmic field of universal love) is the starting point for our world view and comes before our notion of each of us as separate from this larger cosmos and from each other.

Ideas consistent with an evolving world view for nursing science and research were advanced in the nursing literature during the late 1970s and throughout the 1980s and continue to current times, for example, the work of such nursing theorists, researchers, and authors as Davis (1978), Watson (1979, 1981, 1984), Winstead-Fry (1980), Parse (1981), Webster, Jacox, and Baldwin (1981), Downs (1982), Munhall (1982), Chinn (1983), Donaldson (1983), Newman (1979), Leininger (1981), and others currently (Smith & McCarthy, 2010; Watson, 2005; Hills and Watson, 2011).

In general, if one adheres to a human science/caring science perspective, the following areas are acknowledged:

- There is an anomaly between the biological body-physical concept of person in medicine and traditional psychology and the concept of person as a whole referred to in nursing.
- There is a strain between the study of person as a unified *whole* (and human inner subjective experiences/meanings) and the process of nursing care and the traditional reductionistic assumptions of natural science, basic sciences, and biomedical sciences.
- Nursing, in its attempt to mature as a science and profession in its own right, has been susceptible to the temptation to follow the rule of the older natural sciences, medical-clinical views of humans, without clarifying important philosophical, ontological, epistemological, ethical, and scientific questions relevant to the underlying disciplinary foundation for

the study of nursing: human caring, health-illness, healing, and phenomena, which include all the vicissitudes of human existence, sustaining human caring and humanity itself in the world. This disciplinary foundation serves as the moral and scientific covenant nursing has with humankind and society, as the raison d'être of its existence.

Other philosophical and conceptual aspects related to a human science/caring science context for nursing study are as follows:

- Nursing views human beings as evolving, experiencing spiritual beings.
- There is an interconnected evolution of the human consciousness and the global world view shift toward acknowledging the connectedness of all.
- Health is a process and highly subjective as an inner experience.
- Change is ongoing; nurse and person are coparticipants.

A human science perspective allows nursing scholars and researchers to raise serious questions about nursing/caring science and the new directions that nursing must take to be true to its subject matter and its social and scientific responsibility. Moreover, a human caring science perspective opens new vistas and new possibilities for humans and their world of health–illness-healing experiences. Such a perspective allows for the questioning of ultimate meanings and ethical values of humans, health, and nursing.

In summary, a human caring science context is based on the following (Watson, 1984):

- A philosophy of human freedom, choice, and responsibility.
- A biology and psychology of holism (nonreducible persons interconnected with others and nature).
- An expanding and diverse epistemology that allows not only for empirics but for advancement of aesthetics, ethical values, intuition, and process discovery, accommodating all ways of knowing.
- An ontology of time and space.
- A context of interhuman events, processes, and relationships.
- A scientific world view that is open.

It is critical at this point in time that nursing adheres to a perspective that does not disengage nursing's ultimate meanings, intuitions, and relevance from its aesthetics, ethics, science, and practice (Watson, 1984, 1999, 2005, 2008).

In our attempts to be scientific and to advance as a profession and a discipline, we suddenly reached a junction that can lead us in two different directions. One path is that of traditional medical science with its distinctive objective, empirical epistemology. The other path acknowledges nursing as a human caring science with another starting point for its ontological world view, its approach to knowing, knowledge, and epistemology, and its approach to methods (e.g., inviting diverse forms of evolving methods including drama, art, and performance, along with other extant methods such as narrative, story, interpretive forms of inquiry, and others yet to emerge), and thus deepening its approach to professional clinical caring–healing–health practice models.

The traditional science approach is to take the concepts, viewpoints, and techniques of natural science and medicine and apply them to nursing and the lived-in world of human health–illness experiences. To do so, however, we are making certain assumptions about human life and the human caring process in nursing that are nonhuman in character, that is, adopting

- A distinctive epistemology of empirics for evidence and scientific advancement.
- A philosophy of human determinism and control.
- A biology and psychology of organismic–mechanistic physicalism.
- A separatist ontology of space versus time.
- A context of parts, with mind, body, and spirit splits.
- A scientific world view that is closed.
- A methodology of analysis and validation of repetitive facts.

This traditional approach is one in which we accept the position that our fundamental world view is (scientifically) settled and the major responsibility of contemporary nurse practitioners, scholars, and researchers is simply to add to the increasingly complex store of knowledge. This path is haunted by the restricted thinking of the dominant medical science paradigm that labels, categorizes, manipulates, controls, and treats disease; if not disease, then patients, and; if not patients, then persons as objective entitites and variables.

Such an approach is marred by medical scientific values, goals, and interventions laden with paternalistic notions that are inconsistent with nursing and human caring and the notion of a person as an end in and of him- or herself. If the discipline of nursing operates under the traditional approach, it adopts the ethic of empirical science as the hierarchy of "evidence." This ethic of science is recognized by nursing's adherence to a research tradition that concentrates on objectivity, facts, measurement of smaller and smaller parts, and issues of instrumentality, reliability, validity, and operationalization to the extent that nursing is in danger of exhausting the meaning, relevance, and understanding of the values, ethics, goals, and actions that it espouses in its heritage, ideals, and its covenant with humanity. Such a position can disengage nursing's ultimate meanings and intuitions from its aesthetics, ethics, science, and practice. It is limited by its starting point and fundamental scientific and philosophical restrictions of human life and evolving human consciousness.

On the other hand, if we view nursing as a human caring science, we get to cocreate, combine, integrate, and transform our views of science, restoring unitary notions of beauty, art, ethics, and aesthetics of the human-to-human care process, and even love back into nursing. Human caring science is based on an epistemology that can include metaphysics as well as aesthetics, the humanities, art, and empirics as part of clinical sciences.

At this historic 100-year era of modern nursing (2010 is the centenary of Nightingale's life), nursing can and must rediscover its more meaningful ethical-philosophical foundation based on human, even spiritual values, rather than on nonhuman values—returning to our roots to find and establish our own foundation for the future. Nightingale was clear that nursing is a "calling" and is a spiritual practice.

As a human science, rather than a traditional science, nursing can view human life as a gift to be cherished—a process of wonder, awe, miracles, and mystery. Nurses can choose methods that allow for the subjective, inner world of personal meanings of nurse and other. We can choose to study the inner world of experiences rather than the outer world of evidence and observation alone. We can choose to be a part of our method and involved in the clinical research process rather than to be distant, objectively remote, and primarily concerned with the product and process of science. We can choose to pursue more of the private, intimate world of human caring and healing and inner subjective human experiences rather than concentrate on the public world of nonhuman techno-cure techniques and outer behavior.

This different path can expand our limited thinking and allow us, as professionals and scholars, to develop new pictures of what it means to be human, to be a nurse, to be ill, to be healed, and to give and receive human care. Whether we, as nurses, see human life one way or the other is the result of different intentional acts; moreover, how we choose leads us in very different directions and has very different consequences for our practice, our science, *and* our methodology and our personal/professional ways of being in the world. Indeed, our choice has consequences for nursing's contribution to society in the preservation of humanity.

For example, in the early views of R. D. Laing (1965), Scottish psychiatrist, we can choose to see another as a biological organism, and without that person changing or doing anything differently, we can choose to see the person as whole being, like one's self. However, if we are interested in learning about the other as fully human, not a biological organism alone, to begin with a biological view starting point, it is like trying to make ice by boiling water. We cannot get there.

So too if we want a human caring science for our practices and our service to humankind and use the medical–clinical lens to attend to unitary human and human caring, healing, health phenomena, we cannot get there with medicine's starting point for our science and theories and practices.

Perhaps nursing can learn from the wisdom and experience of Sigmund Koch, an eminent theoretical scholar in psychology and the author of *Psychology: A Study of Science* (1959). After a 30-year career devoted to the exploration of the conditions for psychology to become a scientific enterprise, he concluded: "Psychology cannot be a coherent science" (1969, p. 64) . . . psychology has been misconceived . . . and the end result is a syndrome of modern scholarship . . . called *ameaningful thinking, that is, having the same force as the a in words like amoral . . . knowledge as the result of 'processing', rather than discovery.* Koch (1969, p. 64, 65) lamented that psychology must be discovered anew wherein it is established on a more meaningful philosophical foundation. Nursing is in danger of a similar demise if we do not seriously question our scientific approach. Nursing today has room for more optimism if we proceed with caution and stop emulating the medical sciences. We still have time to rediscover our commitments to humans, to humanity, and to human caring and healing processes and establish a more meaningful philosophical foundation from which to proceed.

These new foundations for nursing are grounded in a professional human caring process that connects with and becomes a part of the lived world of human experiences and the inner meaning associated with healing, well-being, health, treatments, and illness. Nursing's maturity is related to questioning the position that the fundamental world view is settled and participating in the cocreation of a new world view that is already emerging in the global field of human evolution. Thus, we help to create a new context for exploring the unique subject matter and the human nature of our science and practices, and for discovering new and diverse methods that are credible, meaningful, and true to our human caring–healing phenomena and a unitary view of humanity and science alike.

NEW DIRECTIONS FOR THE FUTURE

More and more nursing theories and researchers are now beginning to posit a new nursing research tradition that is giving rise to Kuhn's (1969, 1996) common notion of a scientific revolution. There is greater acknowledgment and public recognition that continued adherence to a medical model for nursing practice, and adherence to a traditional natural science model for nursing science is not adequate for addressing the phenomena of human caring in nursing and inner human experiences to actual or potential health problems.

As nursing continues its quest for scientific development, it is through graduate nursing education and theory development, along with exploration of the history and philosophy of science, that nursing has the opportunity to explore its own heritage; become recommitted to nursing values, goals, and philosophies; and explore research methods and options consistent with prevailing views about the nature of nursing. In so doing, nursing scholars and clinicians can continue to critique and admit openly that an inconsistency or anomaly has existed and continues to exist between the medical tradition and/or natural science paradigm and the nature of nursing. Furthermore, such a dilemma has facilitated nursing researchers and theorists to pursue more actively alternative approaches to developing nursing science. Advanced study in nursing is providing nursing scholars with an opportunity to set forth a paradigm about persons-health-environment and human caring processes of nursing different from the medical and natural science paradigm. In addition, nursing is investigating alternative methods for researching nursing phenomena, ironically alongside a resurgence of conventional empirical evidence searches.

As nursing science begins to make a mature paradigmatic shift toward human caring science as its disciplinary foundation or the study of nursing phenomena, it can be argued that there are some major differences in various assumptions underlying conventional science and human caring science. Figure 2-1 provides different assumptions about the nature of reality, the nature of the inquirer-subject-object relationship, and the nature of truth statements.

These differences have been identified by Giorgi (1970b), Marton and Svensson (1979), Marton (1978), Cook and Reichardt (1979a), Watson (2005, 2008, 2011), and others and hold much promise for nursing science. These differences are acknowledged throughout this book.

The traditional science medical paradigm and the human caring science/nursing paradigm differ as shown in Figure 2-1. Cook and Reichardt (1979b) characterize such paradigmatic differences as methodologically linked, but they should not be viewed as mutually exclusive but rather once again as a dialect. Table 2-1 lists different attributes of the dialectic dance of the different paradigms.

Another way of viewing these paradigms is to consider the various dimensions in a paradigm as a continuum, wherein there is movement away from or toward one end of the continuum to the other, depending on one's starting point, assumptions, views of science, nature of the phenomena under study, and so on. Figure 2-2 represents the movement of various dimensions from one stand toward another, without proposing that they are mutually exclusive and always antagonistic. Figure 2-2 does, however, indicate that as nursing seeks to pre-

Figure 2-1   Assumptions underlying nursing science.

	Traditional Science Medical Paradigm	Human Caring Science Nursing Paradigm
Perspective	Objectivity, observational—measurable	Experiential—subjective, metaphysical
Description	Quantitative	Qualitative or combination qualitative/quantitative
Conceptualization	Generalizable	Contextual
Relations	External—often statistically inferred	Internal—person confirmed
Comprehensions	Explanation—prediction	Understanding
Emphasis	Facts—data	Meaning
Use	Technical, validation of knowledge, extension of existing knowledge	Emancipatory—(new insights, theory, discovery, new knowledge)
Structure	Paradigm adherence	Paradigm transcending

Source: Adapted from Guba, E. G., & Lincoln, Y. S. Epistemological and methodological bases of naturalistic inquiry. *Educational Communicaton and Technology Journal* (1982). 30, 2–7.

serve the concept and context of whole person, relational caring, and human caring–healing as part of its scientific phenomena, there will tend to be movement toward expanding and evolving combination approaches in developing nursing as a human caring science.

The issue in nursing science of the present and the future is beyond method and paradigm per se but rather is based on one's world view and predisposes one to see the world and the events within it in profoundly different ways.

In brief, the prevailing world view of extant nursing theory is more and more cosmological, metaphysical, existential, spiritual, phenomenological, inductive, subjective, process-pattern oriented, transpersonal/transcendent, energetically based, and evolving. Because nurses see the world in different ways from the medical–natural science paradigm, nursing theorists and researchers use different methods of inquiry. The differing paradigms of medicine and nursing are not mutually exclusive, but they do represent two different ends of a continuum. As nursing science continues to shift its emphasis and transcend existing paradigms, there are different lenses a nurse can use to approach the perception of nursing as a human caring science.

Table 2-1   Attributes of the Qualitative and Quantitative Paradigms

Qualitative Paradigm	Quantitative Paradigm
Advocates the use of qualitative methods	Advocates the use of quantitative methods
Phenomonologism and verstehen: "concerned with understanding human behavior from the actor's own frame of reference."	Logical-positivism: "seeks the facts or causes of social phenomena with little regard for the subjective states of individuals."
Naturalistic and uncontrolled observation	Obtrusive and controlled measurement
Subjective	Objective
Close to the data; the insider perspective	Removed from the data; the outsider perspective
Grounded, discovery-oriented, exploratory, expansionist, descriptive, and inductive	Ungrounded, verification-oriented, confirmatory, reductionist, inferential, and hypotheticodeductive.
Process-oriented	Outcome-oriented
Valid: real, rich, and deep data	Reliable: hard and replicable data
Ungeneralizable; single case studies	Generalizable; multiple case studies
Holistic	Particularistic
Assumes a dynamic reality	Assumes a stable reality

Source: Adapted from Marton and Svensson (1979, p. 484).

Some of the critical ontological, epistemological, ethical, esthetic, and methodological and professional practice questions still are in need of further exploration. What conditions facilitate and sustain the person as an end, not a means, to some scientific or medical end? What conditions sustain human caring in instances of threatened humanity, biological or otherwise?

For example, nursing is caught in an ontological, moral, ethical-philosophical dilemma. That is, first, nursing and nurses are faced with a situation whereby a person is reduced to a patient. Second, the patient is reduced to the body physical. Finally, the body physical gets reduced to machine. Thus, we witness and practice in clinical conditions whereby a whole person is reduced to the moral status of an object. As soon as this happens, it allows clinicians and scientists to

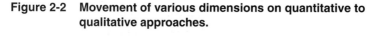

Figure 2-2   Movement of various dimensions on quantitative to qualitative approaches.

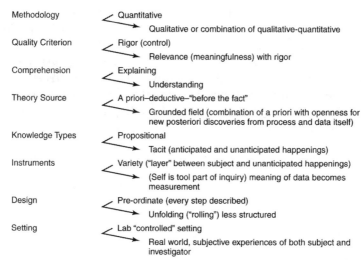

Source: Adapted from Cuba, E. G., & Lincoln, Y. S. (1981). *Effective evaluation: Improving the usefulness of evaluation results through responsive and naturalistic approaches.* San Francisco: Jossey-Bass.

justify doing something to other as object they would not do to a fully functioning person. What we do to another, we likewise impose on ourselves, so we objectify self as we objectify other. This objectification phenomenon is quite dissonant with nursing's values, heritage, orientation, theories, and disciplinary lens.

There is the constant need to critique, to pause, and to reassess nursing practice and science from its core values and disciplinary foundation if nursing is to be sustained as a human caring, healing profession fulfilling its covenant with society. Different variations and differing views affect nursing science and practice and guide methods, helping to determine if a given research method fits the phenomena under study, adhering to methods that sustain humanity and do not diminish the human experience. Generally, nursing phenomena and the human science perspective of nursing are both consistent with the approach that is experiential, qualitative, and contextual. As nursing continues to advance as a human caring science through theory and research, it is called to continue to question its old dogmas, transcend its existing paradigms, and refocus its scientific attention to human phenomena that are consistent with the nature of nursing and preservation of humanity. Nursing scholars are invited to awake to the need to seek out alternative methodologies that lead to increased understanding and contribute new human caring knowledge that is internally relevant for humans. In doing so, nursing has a great potential to contribute to the new knowledge needed to sustain and expand an ethical approach to human caring science and ensure itself a place in academic and scientific circles as a scholarly caring–healing–health discipline worthy of advanced studies, independent practice, and epistemic endeavors that serve society. Nursing has consistently been affirmed by the public as ethical and worthy of public trust. Nursing's evolving science, theories, methods, and practices are expected to adhere to this public vision and hope for survival with integrity and purpose for this century and beyond.

> *"Healing is not a science, but the intuitive art of wooing nature."*
>
> —AUDEN, *THE ART OF HEALING*

REFERENCES

Benner, P., Sutphen, M., Leonard, V., & Day, L. (2010). *Educating nurses: A call for radical transformation. The Carnegie Report for the Advancement of Teaching.* San Francisco: Jossey-Bass.

Boykin, A. & Schoenhofer, S. (2001). *Nursing as caring: A model for transforming practice.* New York: National League for Nursing.

Chinn, P. (1983). Editorial. *Advances in Nursing Science, 5*(2), xi.

Cook, T., & Reichardt, C. (Eds.). (1979a). *Qualitative and quantitative method on evaluation research* (vol. 1, p. 10). Beverly Hills, CA: Sage.

Cook, T., & Reichardt, C. (Eds.). (1979b). *Qualitative and quantitative method on evaluation research* (vol. 1, pp. 9–18). Beverly Hills, CA: Sage.

Davis, A. (1978). The phenomenological approach in nursing research. In N. Chaska (Ed.), *The nursing profession: Views through the mist* (pp. 186–196). New York: McGraw-Hill.

Donaldson, S. (1983). Let us not abandon the humanities. *Nursing Outlook, 31,* 40–43.

Downs, F. S. (1982). It's a great idea—But it won't work. *Nursing Research, 31,* 4.

Giorgi, A. (1970a). *Psychology as a human science* (p. 20). New York: Harper & Row.

Giorgi, A. (1970b). *Psychology as a human science* (pp. 40–56). New York: Harper & Row.

Goodrich, A. (1973). *The social and ethical significance of nursing.* New Haven, CT: Yale University School of Nursing. [Originally published 1915.]

Henderson, V. (1964). The nature of nursing. *American Journal of Nursing, 64,* 62–68.

Hills, M., & Watson, J. (2011). *Creating a caring science curriculum: An emancipatory pedagogy for nursing.* New York: Springer.

Johnson, R. (1975). *In quest of a new psychology* (pp. 18–19). New York: Human Sciences Press.

Koch, S. (1959). *Psychology: A study of science*. New York: McGraw-Hill.

Koch, S. (1969). Psychology cannot be a coherent science. *Psychology Today, 3*(4), 14, 64–68.

Kuhn, T. (1969, 1996). *The structure of scientific revolutions*. (3rd ed.). Chicago: University of Chicago.

Laing, R. D. (1965). *The divided self*. Middlesex, England: Penguin Books.

Leininger, M. (Ed.). (1981). *Caring*. Thorofare, NJ: Charles B. Slack.

Levinas, E. (1969). *Totality and infinity*. Pittsburgh, PA: Duquesne University. (14th printing, 2000).

Marton, F. (1978). *Describing conceptions of the world around us. Reports from the Institute of Education*. Goteborg, Sweden: University of Goteborg.

Marton, F., & Svensson, L. (1979). Conceptions in research in student learning. *Higher Education, 8*, 471–486.

Munhall, P. L. (1982). Nursing philosophy and nursing research: In apposition or opposition? *Nursing Research, 31*, 176–177.

Newman, M. (1979). *Theory development in nursing*. Philadelphia: F. A. Davis.

Newman, M., Sime, A. M., Corcoran-Perry, S. A. (1991). The focus of the discipline of nursing. *Advances in Nursing Science. 13*, 1–14.

Nightingale, F. (1860). *Notes on nursing: What it is and what it is not* (p. 355). New York: Appleton.

Nightingale, F. (1869). In B. M. Dossey, *Florence Nightingale: Mystic, visionary, healer*. (2000). Springerhouse, PA: Springhouse Corporation.

Parse, R. R. (1981). *Man-living health: A theory of nursing*. New York: Wiley.

Smith, M., & McCarthy, P. (2010). Disciplinary knowledge in nursing education: Going beyond the blueprints. *Nursing Outlook, 58*, 44–51.

Watson, J. (1979). *Nursing: The philosophy and science of caring* (pp. 205–215). Boston: Little, Brown.

Watson, J. (1981). Nursing's scientific quest. *Nursing Outlook, 29*(7), 413–416.

Watson, J. (1984). Reflections on new methodologies for study of human care. In M. Leininger (Ed.), *Qualitative methodologies in nursing*. New York: Grune & Stratton.

Watson, J. (2005). *Caring science as sacred science*. Philadelphia: F. A. Davis.

Watson, J. (2008). *Nursing: The philosophy and science of caring* (rev. ed.). Boulder, CO: University Press of Colorado.

Watson, J. (2011). *Postmodern nursing and beyond*. New issue. Boulder, CO: Watson Caring Science Institute.

Watson, J., & Smith, M. (2002). Caring science and the science of unitary human beings. A transtheoretical discourse. *Journal of Advanced Nursing. 37*(5), 452–461.

Webster, G., Jacox, A., & Baldwin, B. (1981). Nursing theory and the ghost of the received view. In J. McCloskey & H. Grace (Eds.), *Current issues in nursing* (pp. 26–34). Boston: Blackwell Publishing.

Winstead-Fry, P. (1980). The scientific method and its impact on holistic health. *Advances in Nursing Science, 2*, 1–7.

BIBLIOGRAPHY

Abdellah, F. G. (1969). The nature of nursing science. *Nursing Research, 18,* 390.

Alexandersson, C. (1981). Amadeo Giorgi's empirical phenomenology (publication no. 3). Swedish Council for Research in Humanities and Social Sciences, Department of Education, University of Goteborg, Sweden.

Chinn, P. (1983). Editorial. *Advances in Nursing Science, 5*(2), xi.

Cook, T., & Reichardt, C. (Eds.). (1979). *Qualitative and quantitative method on evaluation research* (Vol. 1). Beverly Hills, CA: Sage.

Davis, A. (1978). The phenomenological approach in nursing research. In N. Chaska (Ed.), *The nursing profession: Views through the mist.* New York: McGraw-Hill.

Dennis, N. (1982). New methods for research. Paper presented at Western Australian Institute of Technology, Western Australia, May.

Donaldson, S. (1983). Let us not abandon the humanities. *Nursing Outlook, 31,* 40–43.

Downs, F. S. (1982). It's a great idea—But it won't work. *Nursing Research, 31,* 4.

Flaskerud, J. N., & Halloran, E. (1980). Areas of agreement in nursing theory development. *Advances in Nursing Science, 3,* 1–7.

Gaylin, W. (1976). *Caring.* New York: Knopf.

Giorgi, A. (1970). *Psychology as a human science.* New York: Harper & Row.

Guba, E. G., & Lincoln, Y. S. (1982). Epistemological and methodological bases of naturalistic inquiry. *Educational Communication and Technology Journal, 30,* 233–252.

Hall, L. E. (1964). Nursing—What is it? *Canadian Nurse, 60,* 150–154.

Henderson, V. (1964). The nature of nursing. *American Journal of Nursing, 64,* 62–68.

Hyde, A. (1975–1977). *The phenomenon of caring* (vols. 10–12). American Nursing Foundation. Silver Springs, MD: ANF publication.

Johnson, D. (1978). State of art of theory development in nursing. In National League for Nursing (Ed.), *Theory development, What, why, and how.* New York: National League for Nursing.

Johnson, R. (1975). *In quest of a new psychology.* New York: Human Sciences Press.

King, I. (1971). *Toward a theory for nursing.* New York: Wiley.

Koch, S. (1969). Psychology cannot be a coherent science. *Psychology Today, 3,* 64, 66.

Koch, S. (Ed.). (1959). *Psychology: A study of science.* New York: McGraw-Hill.

Kreuter, F. R. (1957). What is good nursing care? *Nursing Outlook, 5,* 302–305.

Leininger, M. (1969). Conference on the nature of science in nursing. Introduction: Nature of science in nursing. *Nursing Research, 18,* 388–389.

Leininger, M. (1979). Foreword. In J. Watson (Ed.), *Nursing: The philosophy and science of caring.* Boston: Little, Brown.

Leininger, M. (Ed.). (1981). *Caring.* Thorofare, NJ: Charles B. Slack.

Levin, M. (1971). Holistic nursing. *Nursing Clinics of North America, 6*(2), 253–264.

Lincoln, Y. S., & Guba, E. G. (1984). *Understanding and doing naturalistic inquiry.* Beverly Hills, CA: Sage.

Marton, F. (1978). *Describing conceptions of the world around us. Reports from the Institute of Education.* Goteborg, Sweden: University of Goteborg.

Marton, F., & Svensson, L. (1979). Conceptions of research in student learning. *Higher Education, 8,* 471–486.

Mayerhoff, M. (1971). *On caring.* New York: Harper & Row.

McKay, R. (1979). Personal communication. Denver, CO: University of Colorado Health Sciences Center.

Munhall, P. L. (1982). Nursing philosophy and nursing research: In apposition or opposition? *Nursing Research, 31,* 176, 177, 181.

Murphy, J. (Ed.). (1971). *Theoretical issues in professional nursing.* New York: Appleton-Century-Crofts.

Newman, M. (1979). *Theory development in nursing.* Philadelphia: F. A. Davis.

Newman, M., Sime, A. M., Corcoran-Perry, S. A. (1991). The focus of the discipline of nursing. *Advances in Nursing Science. 13,* 1–14.

Nightingale, F. (1860). *Notes on nursing: What it is and what it is not.* New York: Appleton.

Norris, C. M. (Ed.). (1969). *Proceedings, First Nursing Theory Conference.* Kansas City, KS: University of Kansas.

Oiler, C. (1982). The phenomenological approach in nursing research. *Nursing Research, 31,* 178, 181.

Omery, A. (1982). Phenomenology: A method for nursing research. *Advances in Nursing Science,* 5, 49–63.

Parse, R. R. (1981). *Man-living health: A theory of nursing.* New York: Wiley.

Paterson, J. D., & Zderak, L. Y. (1976). *Humanistic nursing.* New York: Wiley.

Peplau, H. (1952). *Interpersonal relations in nursing.* New York: Putnam.

Pickering, M. (1980). Introduction to qualitative research methodology. Paper presented at the meeting of the American Speech-Language and Hearing Association, Detroit, November.

Rist, R. C. (1977). On the relations among educational research paradigms: From disdain to detente. *Anthropology Educational Quarterly, 8,* 42–49.

Rogers, M. (1970). *Theoretical basis of nursing.* Philadelphia: F. A. Davis.

Spicker, S., & Gadow, S. (Eds.). (1980). *Nursing images and ideals.* New York: Springer.

Stevens, B. (1979). *Nursing theory.* Boston: Little, Brown.

Valle, R., & King, M. (1978). *Existential phenomenological alternatives for psychology.* New York: Oxford University Press.

Van Kaam, A. L. (1959). Phenomenological analysis: Exemplified by a study of the experience of being really understood. *Individual Psychology, 15,* 66–72.

Watson, J. (1979). *Nursing: The philosophy and science of caring.* Boston: Little, Brown.

Watson, J. (1981a). Nursing's scientific quest. *Nursing Outlook, 29*(7), 413–416.

Watson, J. (1981b). Professional identity crisis—Is nursing finally growing up? *American Journal of Nursing, 81,* 1488–1490.

Watson, J. (1984). Reflections on new methodologies for study of human care. In M. Leininger (Ed.), *Qualitative methodologies in nursing.* New York: Grune & Stratton.

Webster, G., Jacox, A., & Baldwin, B. (1981). Nursing theory and the ghost of the received view. In J. McClosky & H. Grace, (Eds.), *Current issues in nursing.* Boston: Blackwell.

Winstead-Fry, P. (1980). The scientific method and its impact on holistic health. *Advances in Nursing Science, 2,* 1–7.

Yura, K., & Torres, G. (1975). *Today's conceptual frameworks within baccalaureate nursing programs* (17–25). New York: National League of Nursing.

CHAPTER 3

Human Caring in Nursing

"We need a revolution in human caring, if we are to survive in this millennium."

—ALBERTA PERRETTI, ITALIAN PHILOSOPHER, RESPONSIBLE FOR DEVELOPING AN ETHICAL CHARTER FOR HEALTH CARE FOR ALL OF ITALY, JUNE, 2010, PANEL ON HUMAN CARE ITALY CONGRESSO, TURIN, ITALY

"Whether humanity is to continue and comprehensively prosper on spaceship Earth depends entirely on the integrity of human individuals and not on political and economic systems. The cosmic question has been asked: Are humans a worthwhile-to-universe invention?"

—R. BUCKMINSTER FULLER (FROM THE CONFERENCE ON WORLD AFFAIRS, UNIVERSITY OF COLORADO, APRIL 1983)

"As we examine our truth of Belonging-Being-Knowing and Doing-Caring-Healing work in the world, how can we any longer bear to sustain and perpetuate an empty, hollow model?"

—JEAN WATSON (2005, P. 67)

A human caring science approach to health care is required for nursing practice now and in the future. As the nursing profession advances in the scientific–theoretical arena as well as in the area of humanistic clinical practice, a new model of the nurse is needed. Just as the mind is inseparable from the body, the scholarly activities of nursing should not be divorced from its clinical practice. The new model of nursing for education, research, and practice is that of a scholar–clinician. Likewise, the new wave in health care is an individual approach, directed toward the person that honors and integrates all the parts into a unified and significant whole. Quality nursing and health care today demand a humanistic respect for the functional unity of the human being. The phenomena of health–illness–healing must be approached from a broad conceptual base.

The process of human caring for individuals, families, and groups as well as eco-caring, is a major focus for nursing. This is not only because of the dynamic unity of human-to-human ecological connections but because of the requirements of knowledge, commitment, and human values and of the personal, social, and moral engagement of the nurse in time and space.

RATIONALE FOR CLARIFYING NURSING

In the 1930s and 1940s the United States had begun to recognize an epidemic of stress-related illness and disease in our society. Since then, stress has been linked to both mental and physical disease, for example, depression, general anxiety, alcoholism, drug addiction, and breakdown in normal relations with friends, family, and colleagues. Unrelieved stress can lead to hypertension, coronary disease, migraine and tension headaches, peptic ulcers, renal disease, asthma, and even cancer. Stress is also related to low productivity, absenteeism, general unhappiness, poor self-worth, failure, helplessness, hospitalization, and premature deaths. As diseases and health–wellness issues increasingly shift from infectious bacteria-linked etiologies to tension-linked etiologies, nursing care becomes an urgent primary and secondary preventive concern. All this is confounded by the new rapidly advancing health legislation and healthcare reform in the United States. Current shifts are toward prevention, accommodating pre-conditions, chronic illness, with ultimate shift toward health–wellness coaching, and models of caring–healing practices in and out of institutions and into homes and community programs.

Along with increased knowledge and awareness of stress-related health problems is a rapidly growing body of knowledge and skills associated with stress management, coping mechanisms, and stress-reduction strategies. More recently there are scientific quantum leaps with attention to the "quantum" to inner conditions, energy medicine, nonphysical phenomena, and heart and brain research and findings, shattering previously held views of the body physical and mind-body medicine, now shifting to whole person medicine, integral medicine, and era three (III) thinking for medicine and nursing alike. All these developments and world view shifts are becoming and have to become incorporated into the traditional as well as transformative roles of the nurse. There is a shift toward nurse/nursing as archetype and metaphor for yin healing, acknowledging a human being cannot heal with yang energy alone; toward nurse as artist expressing artistry of human caring and healing, restoring heart and soul and love back into health care, as a sacred science and practice (Watson, 2005, 2011). This shift is moving nurses toward an "ontological design architect" (Watson, 1999, 2011) for transforming self and system into caring–healing centers and "habitats for healing" (Quinn, 1992).

A human science and metaphysical view of nursing is adopted in this book as an attempt to develop further and reflect on the science of nursing, the human caring–healing process, and human-to-human environmental and ecological relations that become increasingly important in the already dominant complex technological healthcare (read as sick care technocure) systems.

We are all aware that nursing in the United States, Canada, and other industrialized countries has become increasingly technological and bureaucratic. Even community health nursing, which historically had more flexibility and autonomy, has become increasingly managerial and supervisory. This reality has left the practitioners dispirited and often in despair, searching their way forward in the midst of the chaos and maze of the impersonal structures and impersonal institutional mandates.

There has been a proliferation of the "curing syndrome" and an adoption of the cure techniques, often without regard to costs. To satisfy the increasingly technological and bureaucratic demands of the system, human caring at the individual and group level has received less and less emphasis in the system. It is becoming increasingly difficult for nursing to sustain its caring ideology in practice (Ray, 1981). Institutions and community health systems alike are organized and administered in a manner that is incongruent with professional human caring. Because of the one-sided perspective of the traditional healthcare (illness–cure) system, caring values of nurses and nursing have become submerged. Furthermore, the concept of a human caring function of the nurse is threatened by technology, machines, the high-intensity pace of management, administration, documentation tasks, and the manipulation of people required to meet the needs of the systems.

Preservation and advancement of human caring is a critical issue for nursing and its ability to survive and part of the transformation of health care in society and systems alike unless it is transformed. The mandate for nursing within science as well as within society is a demand for cherishing the wholeness of human and humanity. It is thus that I regard nursing as a human caring science and the human caring process in nursing as a significant humanitarian, ethical, philosophical, and epistemic endeavor and cultivated practice that contributes to the preservation of humanity.

However, some of the critical ontological, epistemological, scientific, ethical, esthetic, methodological, and even metaphysical questions have yet to be explored, except in limited debates by a handful of nursing scholars committed to building and sustaining the disciplinary foundation for the nursing profession and its future. At the same time, these questions that remain to be explored are related to the nature of the very world view and starting point for the subject matter of human and of humanity in the universe regarding how it is defined or codefined.

Furthermore, what conditions facilitate and sustain a person as an end in and of him- or herself and not as a means to some scientific, medical, nursing, or hospital end? What conditions facilitate or sustain human caring and healing in instances of threatened humanity? Of compromised human dignity? What conditions sustain the integrity of a whole person and human caring in instances of threatened biological–organic states? What nursing conditions collectively facilitate and sustain the preservation of humanity in instances of threatened humanity* for nurse/other practitioner as well as patient?

Nursing as a human caring science and human caring is always threatened and fragile. Because human care and caring require a personal, social, moral, and spiritual engagement of the nurse and a commitment to one's self and other humans, nursing offers the promise of human preservation in society.

What I am as a care provider and a caring person and nurse now is, and must be, connected with what I will be for another in the future. The now of human care and caring shapes the future and the ontology of caring in time and space.

Human caring in nursing is therefore not just an emotion, concern, attitude, or benevolent desire. Caring is the moral ideal of nursing whereby the end is protection, enhancement, and preservation of human dignity (Gadow, 1984). Human caring involves values, a will, and a commitment to care, knowledge, caring actions, and consequences. All of human caring is related to intersubjective human responses to health–illness–healing conditions; a knowledge of health–illness, environmental–personal relations, meaning the nurse caring process; and self-knowledge, which is knowledge of one's power and ways of being in relation to both strengths and limitations.

To quote Mayerhoff (1971, p. 13):

> We sometimes speak as if caring did not require knowledge, as if caring for someone, for example, were simply a matter of good intentions or warm regard. . . . To care for someone, I must know many things. I must know, for example, who the other is, what his powers and limitations are, what his needs are, and what is conducive to his growth; I must know how to respond to his needs and what my own powers and limitations are. Such knowledge is both general and specific.

As such, human caring is an ethical, ontological, and epistemic endeavor that defines both nurse and person and a level of time and space. It requires serious study, reflection, action, and a search for new knowledge and new insights that will help to discover new meanings and understanding of the person and human caring process during health–illness–healing experiences.

Such a search for a new knowledge and understandings of human caring then governs some of the epistemological, ethical, intuitive, esthetic, scientific, and methodological conditions for developing nursing as a human caring science.

---

*These ideas were influenced by Professor Gary Stahl, Department of Philosophy, University of Colorado, Boulder.

Moreover, such world view shifts and epistemic endeavors in nursing will help to shed light on both the nurse and the patient or person as valuable ends in and of themselves who are coactive and coparticipants in the human caring–healing process. It is the interdependent, intersubjective, human-to-human caring–healing relationship process, therefore, that can shape conditions necessary to sustain a person and caring in instances where humanity is threatened.

REFERENCES

Gadow, S. (1984). Existential advocacy as a form of caring: Technology, truth, and touch. Paper presented to the Research Seminar Series: The Development of Nursing as a Human Science. School of Nursing, University of Colorado Health Sciences Center, Denver, March.

Mayerhoff, M. (1971). *On caring*. New York: Harper & Row.

Quinn, J. F. (1992). Holding sacred space: The nurse as healing environment. *Holistic Nursing Practice, 6*(4), 26–35.

Ray, M. (1981). A philosophical analysis of caring within nursing. In M. Leininger (Ed.), *Caring: An essential human need*. Thorofare, NJ: Charles B. Slack.

Watson, J. (2005). *Caring science as sacred science*. Philadelphia: F. A. Davis.

Watson, J. (2011). *Postmodern nursing and beyond* (rev. ed.). Boulder, CO: Watson Caring Science Institute.

BIBLIOGRAPHY

Gadow, S. (1984). Existential advocacy as a form of caring: Technology, truth, and touch. Paper presented to the Research Seminar Series: The Development of Nursing as a Human Science. School of Nursing, University of Colorado Health Sciences Center, Denver, March.

Mayerhoff, M. (1971). *On caring*. New York: Harper & Row.

Ray, M. (1981). A philosophical analysis of caring within nursing. In M. Leininger (Ed.), *Caring: An essential human need*. Thorofare, NJ: Charles B. Slack.

CHAPTER 4

Nature of Human Caring and Caring Values in Nursing

"The only true standard of greatness of any civilization is our sense of social and moral responsibility in translating material wealth to human values and achieving our full potential as a caring society."

—THE RIGHT HONORABLE NORMAN KIRK
(FROM A SPEECH GIVEN BY THE FORMER PRIME MINISTER OF NEW ZEALAND)

In this chapter we discuss the values underlying human caring science in nursing. The basic assumptions related to human caring values are put forth, along with some acknowledgment of the dual nature of the relationship between caring and noncaring.

A recognition and acknowledgment of the value of human caring in nursing comes before and presupposes actual caring. A nurse who performs actions toward a patient out of a sense of duty or moral obligation is an ethical nurse. Yet it may be false to say he or she cared about the patient. The value of human care and caring involves a higher sense of spirit of self. Caring calls for a philosophy of moral commitment toward protecting human dignity and preserving humanity. According to Gaut (1983a), the general family of meanings related to the notion of caring includes individual attention to and concern for; individual responsibility for or providing for at some level; and individual regard, fondness, or attachment.

The ideal and value of caring is clearly not just a thing out there but is a starting point, a stance, an attitude, a consciousness, that becomes an intentional commitment and a will toward "seeing" and being present with loving, caring consciousness manifesting in concrete doing and being. Human caring, as a moral ideal, also transcends the action itself and goes beyond the specific act of an individual nurse. Therefore, individually and collectively the nursing profession has a role to play in offering and sustaining collective acts of caring that have important consequences for human civilization.

The essence of the value of human care and caring may be futile unless it contributes to a philosophy of action. Gaut (1983b) goes further and says the action must be judged solely on the welfare of the person being cared for.

The actual concrete action of caring can transcend the value (and pass it on). Embedded in this idea is the notion that caring values and actions can be contagious, at an individual and systemic level, if sufficient conditions are met.

The value of caring is grounded in the self-transcending creative nurse. Gaut (1983c) indicates the following as the necessary and sufficient conditions for caring:

- Awareness and knowledge about one's need for care
- An intention to act, and actions based on knowledge
- A positive change as result of caring, judged solely on basis of welfare of others

I would add that there must be an underlying value, an evolved consciousness, an intentionality and moral commitment to caring for self and other along with a will to care.

For nursing to be truly responsive to the needs of society and make contributions that are consistent with its roots and early origins, both nursing education and the healthcare delivery system need to be based on human values and concern for the welfare of others. Caring outcomes in practice, research, and theory depend on the teaching of a caring ethic, a philosophical orientation toward honoring the whole person and all of humanity, along with knowledge and skills of caring both in one's ways of being as well as in practicing and living out caring modalities, all based on a caring science orientation toward professional practice. As the human threats from biotechnology, scientific engineering, fragmented treatment, bureaucracy, economic mandates, and depersonalization continue to increase and spread in our healthcare delivery system, so must we increase and radiate the human caring philosophy, knowledge, and practices in our system.

The nursing profession has an ethical and social responsibility to both individuals and society to sustain human caring in instances where it is threatened and to be the guardian of human caring, individually and collectively, serving as the vanguard of society's human caring needs now and in the future. If nursing does not fulfill its societal mandate for sustaining human caring, preserving human dignity and humanness in self, systems, and society, it will not be carrying out its covenant to humankind and its reason for existence as a profession.

The following are assumptions related to human caring values in nursing (Watson, 2008):

1. Human caring and love are the most universal, the most tremendous, and the most mysterious of cosmic forces: They comprise the primal and universal psychic energy (de Chardin, 1967a).
2. Often, this wisdom and these needs are overlooked. Although we know people need each other in loving and caring ways, often we do not behave well toward each other. If our humanness and humanity is to survive and

if we are to evolve toward a more loving, moral community and civilization, we need to become more caring and loving to nourish our humanity and evolve as a civilization and live together (de Chardin, 1967b).

3. Because nursing is a caring profession, its ability to sustain its caring ideals, ethics, and philosophy for professional practices affect the human development of civilization and nursing's mission to society. Sustaining a caring ethical ideology affects the human development of civilization and determines nursing's contribution to society.

4. As a beginning we have to learn how to offer caring love, forgiveness, compassion and mercy to ourselves before we can offer authentic caring, tenderness, compassion, love, and dignity to others (de Chardin, 1967c; Watson, 2008).

5. Nursing has always held a human care and caring stance with respect to people and their health–illness–healing concerns.

6. Knowledgeable, informed, and ethical human caring is the essence of professional nursing values, commitments, and competent actions. It is the most central and unifying source to sustain its covenant to society and ensure its survival (Leininger, 1981).

7. Human caring, at the individual and group level, has received less and less emphasis in the healthcare delivery system but now has to be restored if systems are to survive as ethically and scientifically responsible to society and if nursing is to survive as a distinct profession fulfilling its social mandate.

8. Caring values of nurses and nursing have been submerged. Nursing and society are therefore in a critical situation today in sustaining human caring ideals and a caring ideology in practice. The human care role is threatened by increased medical, technological, economic, bureaucratic, and managerial institutional constraints in this post post–modern era of dramatic and chaotic unprecedented change in human history. At the same time there has been a proliferation of radical treatment and cure techniques, often without regard to costs to human existence or outcomes for individuals and the public at large.

9. Preservation and advancement of human caring as an ethical, philosophical, epistemic, and clinical endeavor are significant issues for nursing today and in the future.

10. Human caring can be most effectively demonstrated and practiced only interpersonally. The intersubjective human process keeps alive a common sense of humanity; it teaches us how to be human by identifying ourselves with others, whereby the humanity of one is reflected in

the other. However, caring consciousness can transcend time, space, and physicality and affect the evolving consciousness of humanity at large (Watson, 2008, 2011).

11. Nursing's social, moral, professional, and scientific contributions to humankind and society lie in its commitment to sustain and advance human caring values, knowledge, practices, and ideals in theory, practice, education, and research.

CARING AND NONCARING

It is important to notice the dual nature of the relation between caring and noncaring. What we call caring on one occasion must be the same as what we call caring on another occasion. Nursing sets before itself an ideal that it is trying to reach. Caring must be the same thing that one achieves at one moment when one is caring or fails to achieve when one fails to be caring.

We can also approach caring by the method of contrast. A distinction can be found in society (and in nursing) in some form between those persons (nurses) who are caring and those who are uncaring. The most abstract characteristics of a caring person is that he or she is somehow responsive to a person as a unique individual, perceives the other's feelings, and sets apart one person from another from the ordinary. The uncaring person is by contrast insensitive to another person as a unique individual, not perceptive of the other's feelings, and does not necessarily distinguish one person from another in any significant way.

Early empirical research on caring in nursing substantiated the above view that caring indeed connotes a personal response. The early findings of Watson et al. (1979) derived caring categories from empirical data that revealed the following processes:

- treating the individual as a person,
- concern and empathy,
- personalized characteristics of the nurse,
- communication process, and
- extra effort.

Moreover, Watson's 1983 cross-cultural data on caring in nursing supports some of the above findings. A study of human caring among Australian Anglo Saxons and Aborigines and Chinese in Taiwan revealed strong and consistent results linking caring to personal responses.

The cross-cultural data included categories such as "nurse presence" (including touch) and physical "felt presence" from nurses across time (e.g., sharing an experience across time), "nurse feelings exchanged" (such as exchanging of love, sharing sorrow and pain, and letting a person express feeling), and a category related to caring nurses "giving time and taking time" (this category included follow-up visits, presence, visitation). All these findings are consistent with an individual approach and of conscious acts that convey a will and intention to care, along with specific actions.

Both theoretically and empirically the concept of caring is not merely characterized by certain categories or classes of nursing actions but as ideals and directions toward desired actions of being and doing. Each instance of human caring and human caring moments exists in a given time and space and can never be repeated in the same way again. What happens in a given moment has consequences for both nurse and patient and informs each other's next moments of caring.

Other classic research on caring and noncaring has been reported elsewhere in my writings but deserves to be included here again, such as the research of Halldorsdottir (1991). These classic findings of clinical research on caring from a patient's experiential view and nurse–patient relationship revealed a continuum from uncaring to caring.

Uncaring can be classified as follows:

- Biocidic: life destroying; leading to anger, despair, and decreased well-being
- Biostatic: life restraining; patient experienced the nurse as cold and treatment as a nuisance
- Biopassive: life neutral; nurse apathetic and detached (just doing the job)

Caring can be classified as follows:

- Bioactive: life sustaining; reflected in the classic nurse–patient relationship and as kind, concerned, benevolent, and responsive
- Biogenic: highest level of human-to-human caring; life giving and life receiving for both nurse and patient

The biocidic to biogenic continuum has relevance to all nurse–patient relationships and can serve as an intellectual, theoretical, and ethical guide toward one's presence with another in any caring occasion. The biogenic caring represents the highest level of caring related to healing, wholeness, and a transpersonal caring relationship in that both nurse and patient are affected by the relationship. To paraphrase Halldorsdottir (1991): Biogenic caring involves a loving presence and a generosity of spirit, mercy, and compassion. A truly life giving presence of being open and giving from the heart, receptive with respect, compassion, and dignity, creating a trusting relationship that is human-to-human.

Such a relationship opens up access to higher dimensions of caring and healing from the source of life itself. Such philosophical and empirical data on caring provide us with ways to contrast caring with noncaring to get a better understanding of the phenomena.

At this point in understanding of the deeper ethic of caring, I consider biocidic and biostatic caring to be unethical. Although we can acknowledge we are all human and some instances of biopassive caring will exist, we can awaken to not perpetuating the biocidic, biostatic, and biopassive modes as part of creating and sustaining a culture of caring for self and system and even society.

WATSON'S VALUE SYSTEM

The value system set forth here regarding a theory of human caring consists of values associated with deep respect for the wonders and mysteries of life and acknowledgment of a spiritual dimension to life and internal power of the human caring process, growth, and change. Human caring requires high regard and reverence for a person and human life, a love of humanity, nonpaternalistic values related to human autonomy, inner wisdom, and freedom of choice. There is a high value on the subjective–internal life world of the experiencing person and how the person (both patient and nurse) is perceiving and experiencing health–illness conditions in the meaning one holds for his or her experience, honoring his or her individual search for meaning that goes beyond the condition or situation itself.

An emphasis is placed on helping a person gain more self-knowledge, self-control, self-caring, and inner healing of self, regardless of the external health condition. The nurse is viewed as a coparticipant in the human caring–healing process. Therefore, a high value is placed on the relationship between nurse and other.

This value system is blended with Watson's 10 carative factors (Watson, 1979, 2008), such as humanistic altruism, practice of heart-centered loving kindness and equanimity, sensitivity to one's self and others, and love for and trust of life and other humans (Table 4-1).

Underlying the value system is a call for a revaluing of humans and human caring in theory, education, practice, and science—thus a rationale for developing nursing as a human caring science wherein the human–universe connection is the starting point. Such a perspective leads to some metaphysical considerations that are necessary to discuss before moving forward.

Table 4-1 Watson's Original 10 Carative Factors and Refined Carative Processes

Original Carative Factors (Watson, 1979)	Refined Carative Processes (Watson, 2008)
1. Humanistic–altruistic system of values	Practice of loving–kindness/compassion and equanimity with self/other
2. Enabling faith–hope	Being authentically present; enabling belief system and subjective world of self/other
3. Cultivation of sensitivity to self and others	Cultivating own spiritual practices; beyond ego-self to authentic transpersonal presence
4. Helping–trusting, human care relationship	Sustaining a loving, trusting, and caring relationship
5. Expressing positive and negative feelings	Allowing for expression of feelings; authentically listening and "holding another person's story for them"
6. Creative problem-solving caring process	Creative solution seeking through caring process, full use of self; all ways of knowing/ doing/being; engage in artistry of human caring–healing practices and modalities
7. Transpersonal teaching–learning	Authentic teaching–learning within context of caring relationship; stay within other's frame of reference; shift toward a health–healing– wellness coaching model
8. Supportive, protective, and/or corrective mental, physical, societal, and spiritual environment	Creating healing environment at all levels; physical/ nonphysical, subtle environment of energy, consciousness, wholeness, beauty, dignity, and peace are potentiated
9. Human needs assistance	Reverentially and respectfully assisting with basic needs, holding an intentional, caring consciousness of touching the embodied spirit of another as sacred practice, working with life force/life energy/life mystery of another
10. Existential–phenomenological– spiritual forces	Opening and attending to spiritual, mysterious, unknown, and existential dimensions of all the vicissitudes of life, death, suffering, pain, joy, transitions life change; "allowing for a miracle." All of this is presupposed by a knowledge base and clinical competence.

Source: Watson, J. (2008). Nursing. *The philosophy and science of caring.* (Rev. Ed.). Boulder, CO: University Press of Colorado. Reprinted by permission. University Press of Colorado.

REFERENCES

de Chardin, T. (1967). *On love* (pp. 7–8). New York: Harper & Row.

Gaut, D. (1983). Development of a theoretically adequate description of caring. *Western Journal of Nursing Research, 5*(4), 313–324.

Halldorsdottir, S. (1991). Five basic modes of being with another. In D. A. Gaut & M. Leininger (Eds.), *Caring: The compassionate healer.* New York: National League for Nursing Press.

Leininger, M. (Ed.). (1981). *Caring: An essential human need.* Thorofare, NJ: Charles B. Slack.

Watson, J. (1979). *Nursing: The philosophy and science of caring* (pp. 9–10). Boston: Little, Brown.

Watson, J. (1983). Caring and loss-grieving experiences. New knowledge for nursing practice. Research presented at the American Nurses Association Clinical and Scientific Sessions. Denver, CO, November.

Watson, J. (2008). *Nursing. The philosophy and science of caring.* (Revised Ed.). Boulder, CO: University Press of Colorado.

Watson, J. (2011). *Postmodern nursing and beyond* (rev. ed.). Boulder, CO: Watson Caring Science Institute.

Watson, J., Burckhardt, C., Brown, I., Bloch, D., & Hester, N. (1979). A model of caring. In the *American Nurses Association, Clinical and Scientific Sessions* (pp. 32–44). Editor ANA Kansas City, MO: American Nurses Association.

BIBLIOGRAPHY

de Chardin, T. (1967). *On love* (pp. 7–8). New York: Harper & Row.

Gaut, D. (1983). Development of a theoretically adequate description of caring. *Western Journal of Nursing Research, 5*(4), 313–324.

Leininger, M. (Ed.). (1981). *Caring: An essential human need.* Thorofare, NJ: Charles B. Slack.

Watson, J. (1979). *Nursing: The philosophy and science of caring* (pp. 9–10). Boston: Little, Brown.

Watson, J. (1983). Caring and loss-grieving experiences. New knowledge for nursing practice. Research presented at the American Nurses Association Clinical and Scientific Sessions. Denver, CO, November.

Watson, J., Burckhardt, C., Brown, I., Bloch, D., & Hester, N. (1979). A model of caring. In the *American Nurses Association, Clinical and Scientific Sessions* (pp. 32–44). Editor ANA. Kansas City, MO: American Nurses Association.

CHAPTER 5

Nursing and Metaphysics

"Still another such need, strangely, is the need for metaphysics herself,
. . . What am I? What is death—and more puzzling still, what is birth?
A beginning? An ending? . . . does it matter?"

—RICHARD TAYLOR (1974, P. 6)

The previous chapters attempted to set forth a view of nursing that is consistent with nursing's tradition of human caring rather than the tradition of medicine. In advancing such a view there is a call for a revaluation of humans and caring. The alternative world view of nursing that is being suggested will place nursing within a metaphysical context and establish nursing as a human-to-human caring process with spiritual dimensions rather than a set of behaviors that conform to the traditional science/medical model.

Western science, psychology, and even nursing have dealt very poorly with the spiritual side of human nature; it is either ignored or labeled pathological, too religious, too abstract, too extreme, or controversial. Yet much of the agony of our time stems from a spiritual vacuum. Western culture and our study of people and nursing has ruled out spiritual nature, but the cost is great (Tart, 1976).

A metaphysical context becomes important not only to me in my writing, but my context gives the reader a better perspective of my values and beliefs and the opportunity to assess how these mesh with my ideas and with one's own ideas. It also becomes useful for any nurse, whether he or she is a scholar, teacher, researcher, or practitioner of nursing, to step back and examine nursing as a professional, social, and scientific endeavor that exists as a compassionate service to humankind. As such, it is necessary to examine and reflect on what nursing is, does, stands for, and could or should contribute to society.

The questions beyond the starting point of my ideas are these: What should nursing be about? What change of values, goals, and visions are required for nursing to actualize its true sense of direction, its true moral, social and scientific contribution? What lens change is necessary? What point of view needs examining? Does any of this require a new starting point, or do we need greater lens power "to see" or "to be"? All of this, of course, fits within a broader context of society, environment, culture, politics, time, space, the universe, and the cosmos itself.

My nursing views are of the ideal of what may be or can be rather than what is. However, they also acknowledge that what exists as the essence and power of nursing is underdeveloped and often overlooked.

ROLE OF METAPHYSICS IN WESTERN SCIENCE

Most people today are aware that with the rise of natural sciences throughout the history and philosophy of science, the positivistic-reductionist approach dominated Western science and medicine and affected nursing. Progressive thinkers who incorporated metaphysical beliefs into their ideas were often disregarded or rejected. Because of the positivist tradition of Western science and the advancement of medical science, Eastern thought that incorporated the spiritual aspect of humanness has had little impact on nursing. However, Eastern ideas and philosophies are very common in the writings of different 19th and early 20th century poets and authors, including such transcendentalists as Ralph Waldo Emerson, Henry David Thoreau, Walt Whitman, and to some extent William James. Even Florence Nightingale offered a metaphysical orientation when she emphasized that nature restored and preserved health. In essence, the nurse was to be good and loving; "go your way straight to God's work in simplicity and singleness of heart" (Nightingale, 1860, p. 76). Nightingale was also clear that nursing is a spiritual practice. Other early historians of nursing posited that the principal condition in human survival is human caring (Dock & Stewart, 1920).

Among modern theorists, C. G. Jung certainly had a strong orientation toward Eastern thought and religions. Jung (1968) talked about people facing their souls. So while the 19th century writers and poets glimpsed "cosmic consciousness" (a phrase Walt Whitman borrowed from Vedantic philosophy of India [Hall & Lindsay, 1978]), only more recently have these ideas been of interest to Western thinkers and scientists and nurses.

Medical science has moved from an integrated approach in the early stages— the physician as healer and priest era (where the mind, body, and soul were united for care and cure)—to the period of scientism where they split apart and different specialists, different healthcare providers, or different technologies or medical treatments were applied to the different components of the person. In the current period the person is split further and further apart and the soul is either replaced with narcissism of self or denied altogether. The human soul is further destroyed with a depersonalized, artificial environment, advanced technology, and robotic, even biocidic, treatment for cure, delivered by strangers in a strange environment.

The developmental trends of humankind throughout history indicate that an awareness of psychological or mental processes, an evolving human consciousness, comes about more slowly than an awareness of physical concerns. Just as history seems to repeat itself, movements tend to be evolutionary rather than revolutionary, cyclical, and spiral. Take, for example, the idea of "self," which is a relatively recent term in psychology. Although some late 18th century and early 20th century literary works were among the first to develop the concept of self (such as those by Jane Austen, Henry James, and William James), the notion of self was picked up later by the more scientific world of psychology and sociology. Perhaps Allport and Maslow in the 1950s and 1960s were the first psychologists really to begin to focus on the notion of self. This was followed by the human potential movement in psychology and related fields exemplified by Carl Rogers, Fritz Perls, the Esalen movement, and so on; all were attempts to uncover, discover, recover, and restore one's sense of self. During the evolution of scientific–philosophical advancements, coupled with the changing world views of what it means to have a self and to be human, nursing has possessed the primary responsibility of caring for people in health and illness. The degree to which the nurse cared for patients and the focus of what was important for caring changed and continued to change. However, the aspect of lasting significance is that nurses cared for and about others.

The thesis of this work is that caring as an intersubjective human–environment–universe process and relationship is the moral ideal of nursing. Nursing therefore has an important societal role in the enhancement of dignity and the preservation of humanity. Indeed, nursing's role in society is based on human caring; its social contribution lies in its moral commitment to human caring. It also has an important humanistic and scientific contribution to make in the field of human sciences and health sciences in pursuing human care as a serious epistemic endeavor. This scientific awareness has been long in coming and slow to be recognized, and still has far to go. Nevertheless, human caring and theory and knowledge can now be viewed as a significant ethical, philosophical, scientific pursuit. Moreover, there is more social, artistic, literary, and scientific freedom and permission to attend to moral and metaphysical matters today than in the 1960s, with its scientism rise. There is now recognition of an inner self, inner resources, acknowledgment of spiritual self, or the need for integration of the mind, body, and soul along with a view of unitary being and of unitary world view. Our concept of human development need not stop with ideas of self and self-actualization but can allow for spiritual awakening and pursuit of harmony of unitary being and mind-body-spirit-soul-universe connection.

It is ironic that in a time of such tangible, factual, scientific, and technological advancement in medical science, we have to turn to some sense of mysterious, intangible, philosophical, and metaphysical, sometimes even mystical, worlds of humans to solve some of the sickness in society, the suffering associated with disharmony with the mind, body, and soul.

As a result of the historical movements, nursing is now at a point where it can also consider some metaphysical and moral ideals as guides for its own efforts. Nursing science can benefit from a metaphysical approach that revalues the higher spiritual sense of being human and links that with human caring as it advances itself as a human caring science for the 21st century. Nursing can in turn help justify its human concern to build a more fully informed understanding of the spiritual realms and where that leads us as humans and scientists.

The nursing theory I continue to develop attempts to make explicit my metaphysical position regarding mind, body, spirit, and soul and to acknowledge how my beginning position on this issue directs my concept of nursing and caring processes. To illustrate the complexities of metaphysical issues that confront nursing, whether they are acknowledged or not, I include here Chapter 1, "The Need for Metaphysics" (pp. 5–9), from Richard Taylor's book, *Metaphysics* (1974). This chapter can be a beginning context for nurses to consider their own views on the complex matter of being and knowing and to learn how it is impossible to escape metaphysics, regardless of how hard one tries or how many substitutes are created. The chapter, which follows, helps one to examine the need for metaphysics that can guide one's response to others and affect nursing theories, practice, and research.

The Need for Metaphysics
Richard Taylor

There are many things one can do without. Among them are even things foolish persons devote their life's energy to winning. One can do without wealth, for example, and be no less happy. One can do without position, status, or power over others, and be no less happy, certainly no less human. Very likely, without these one will be more human, more the kind of being nature or God, whatever gave him being in the first place, intended. Indeed such things as these—possessions, power, notoriety, which mean so much to the unreflective—appear on examination to be no more than desperate attempts to give meaning to a life that is without meaning. They reflect the vain notion that one's worth can be protected, even enhanced, by enough accumulation, if not of gold, then of its modern equivalents. When this fails, the pursuit of such things as often as not becomes little more than the response to the need to have something to do. Few people are able to sit still, much less to sit still and think; and when enforced idleness threatens, most people begin to plan distant places to go to, purchases to be made, or pictures to take in far off lands—in short, something to do. Just the going and coming will keep them busy for a while, get them through that much of life, and take their minds off things by presenting a variety and novelty to their sense organs. Perhaps man is, as the ancients declared, a rational animal; but if this is so, it is only in the sense that he is uniquely capable of reason, contemplation, and thought, not that he spends much of his life at it. We still share with the rest of animate creatures restless needs and cravings that drive us to movement perpetually. Aristotle's dictum that life is motion surely applies to our own lives. It is what we share with other animals that is most apparent, not the elusive qualities that set us apart. The same philosopher associated reason and thought and contemplation with the gods. He did not first look to mortals for the expression of intelligence—except, interestingly, to those few of its specimens gifted with the love for philosophy and metaphysics, and whose happiness he therefore compared to that of the gods.

The Love of Man and of Nature

There are, however, some things one cannot do without, at least not without deep suffering and the diminishing of one's nature. Among these is the love and approbation of at least a few of one's fellows. Lacking these, one seeks the semblance of them in the form of feigned affection, pretended deference, awe, and sometimes fear. It is astonishing that these counterfeits will so often do, will even seem to give significance to people's lives. Yet we see on every side that this is in fact so. The explanation is of course not in the worth of these things themselves, but in the depth of the need people vainly seek to satisfy through the means of such things.

Another need that cannot be destroyed or left unmet without great damage, of which metaphysicians have often been acutely aware, is the love for nature and the feeling of our place within it. Without this we become machines, grinding out our days and hours to that merciful end when death imposes the peace we have never been able to find for ourselves. A child easily thinks of himself as something apart, a virtual center of reality about which the whole of nature turns, to whose wants everything ministers. One who loves nature rises above this paltry conception of his own being and becomes sensitive to his identity with the whole of reality, which is without beginning or end. This partially explains the difficulty many persons have in fathoming metaphysics. It is not that it is so difficult, but that it is approached from the wrong point of view—from a childhood mentality, from the standpoint of one who finds himself always at the center of the stage, all else being a vast thing without spirit or soul. It is hardly the frame of mind in which to understand a Plato, a Buddha, or a Spinoza.

Metaphysics and Wisdom

Still another such need, strangely, is the need for metaphysics herself. We cannot live as fully rational men without her. This does not mean that metaphysics promises the usual rewards that a scientific knowledge of the world so stingily withholds. She does not promise freedom, God, immortality, or anything of the sort. She offers neither a rational hope nor the knowledge of these. Metaphysics in fact promises no knowledge of anything. If knowledge itself is what one seeks, he should be grateful for empirical science, for he will never find it in metaphysics.

Then what is her reward? What does metaphysics offer that is in her power alone to give? What, that this boundless world cannot give even to the richest and most powerful—that she seems, in fact, to withhold from these more resolutely than from the poor and the humble? Her reward is wisdom. Not boundless wisdom, not invincible truth, which must be left to the gods, not a great understanding of the cosmos or of man, but wisdom, just the same; and it is as precious as it is rare.

What, then, is so good about it? What is wisdom worth if it does not fulfill our deep cravings, such as the craving for freedom, for gods to worship, for a bit more of life than material nature seems to promise? What makes it worth seeking at all?

The first reward of such wisdom is, negatively, that it saves one from the numberless substitutes that are constantly invented and tirelessly peddled to the simpleminded, usually with stunning success, because there is never any dearth of customers. It saves us from these glittering gems and baubles, promises and dogmas and creeds that are worth no more than the stones under one's feet. Fools grasp, at the slightest solicitation, for any specious substitute that offers a hope for the fulfillment of their desires, the products of brains conditioned by greed and competition, no matter how stupid, sick, or destructive these may be. Many persons, in response to the deep need to be loved, of which we have spoken, have felt themselves transformed by a mere utterance; such as, for example, "Jesus loves you!", an assurance that is cheaply and insincerely flung at them by an ambitious evangelist. The instant conviction that such banishments sometimes produce is uncritically taken to be a sign of their certain truth, when in fact they signify nothing more than a need which demands somehow to be met, by whatever means. Again, many persons can banish at will, even before it is really felt, the dread and the objective certainty of their own inevitable destruction. For this comfort they need nothing more than the mere reminder of some promise expressed in a text of ancient authority, or some holy book, or even the simple declamation of a clever and manipulative preacher. In this way does the religion of faith, perverting everything and turning the world upside down, serve as the cheap metaphysics, not of the poor, but of those impoverished in spirit and wanting in wisdom, some of whom bask in a blaze of worldly glory. Such religion, substituting empty utterance for thought, is not the religion of the metaphysical mind or of those who love God and nature first and themselves as a reflection of this.

Where religion can make no headway, in the mind of the skeptic, ideology can sometimes offer some sort of satisfaction to much the same need. Thus many persons spend their lives in a sandcastle, a daydream, in which every answer to every metaphysical question decorates its many mansions. The whole thing is the creation of their brains, or worse, of their needs—it is an empty dream, for nothing has been created except illusions. Such dreams are not metaphysics, but the substitute for metaphysics. They illustrate again how one can live without metaphysics only if some substitute, however specious, is supplied, and this is testimony to the deep need for her.

What am I? What is this world, and why is it such? Why is it not like the moon— bleak, barren, hostile, meaningless? How can such a thing as this be? What is this brain; does it think? And this craving or will, whence does it arise? Is it free? Does it perish with me, or not? Is it perhaps everlasting? What is death—and more puzzling still, what is birth? A beginning? An ending? And life—is it a clock- work? Does the world offer no alternatives? And if so, does it matter? What can one think about the gods, if anything at all? Are there any? Or is nature herself her own creator, and the creator of me; both cradle and tomb, both holy and mundane, both heaven and hell?

The answers to such things are not known. They never will be. It is pointless to seek the answers in the human brain, in science, or in the pages of philosophy and metaphysics. But they will be sought, just the same, by everyone who has a brain, by the stupid as well as the learned, by the child, the man, by whoever can look at the world with wonder. False and contrived answers will always abound. There will always be those who declare that they know the answers to these things, that they "found" these answers in some religious experience, in some esoteric book of "divine" authorship, or in something occult. They do not find them; they find nothing at all except the evaporation of their need to go on asking questions, and of their fears of what the answers to those questions could turn out to be. They find, in other words, a comfort born of ignorance.

So the need of metaphysics endures. No one will shake it off. Metaphysics will be shunned by most people, always, because her path is not easy and no cer- tain treasures lie at the end. Her poor cousins will be chosen in preference, because they offer everything at no cost—a god to worship who has set us apart from the rest of creation and guarantees each an individual immortality, and a will that is free to create a destiny.

People will always choose substitutes for metaphysics. Because of the inde- structible need for her, they will accept anything, however tawdry, however absurd, as a surrogate. Yet it is only metaphysics that, while preserving one in the deepest ignorance, while delivering up not the smallest grain of knowledge of anything, will nevertheless give that which alone is worth holding to, repudiating whatever promises something better. For metaphysics promises wisdom, a wisdom sometimes inseparable from ignorance, but whose glow is nevertheless genuine, from itself, not borrowed, and not merely the reflection of our bright and selfish hopes.

Because of the nature of this text, with its emphasis on humans and human caring in nursing, it is inevitable that there are metaphysical overtones. When a discipline's primary subject matter is tied to humans, life, death, and such abstract notions as health, illness, and human care processes, it is impossible to limit ideas strictly to empirical sciences and the physical–materialistic view of life.

One also seeks some greater, deeper reflection, explanations, meanings, and sense of wisdom that goes beyond the knowledge, facts, and external events per se. As such, it is necessary to be forthright about one's metaphysical beliefs; human life, then, becomes the foundation of my ideas about nursing as a deeply human activity.

REFERENCES

Dock, L., & Stewart, I. M. (1920). *A short history of nursing* (vol. 1). New York: Putnam.

Hall, C. S., & Lindsay, G. (1978). *Theories of personality* (3rd ed., p. 351). New York: Wiley.

Jung, C. G. (1968). Psychology and alchemy. In H. Read, M. Fordham, & G. Adler (Eds.), *Collected works of C.G. Jung* (vol. 12, pp. 99–101). Princeton, NJ: Princeton University Press.

Nightingale, F. (1860). *Notes on nursing: What it is and what it is not* (pp. 135–136). New York: Appleton.

Tart, C. (Ed.). (1976). *Transpersonal psychologies*. New York: Harper & Row.

Taylor, R. (1974). *Metaphysics* (2nd ed., pp. 5–9). Englewood Cliffs, NJ: Prentice-Hall.

BIBLIOGRAPHY

Dock, L., & Stewart, I. M. (1920). *A short history of nursing* (vol. 1). New York: Putnam.

Hall, C. S., & Lindsay, G. (1978). *Theories of personality* (3rd ed.). New York: Wiley.

Jung, C. G. (1968). Psychology and alchemy. In H. Read, M. Fordham, & G. Adler (Eds.), *Collected works of C. G. Jung* (vol. 12). Princeton, NJ: Princeton University Press.

Nightingale, F. (1860). *Notes on nursing: What it is and what it is not.* New York: Appleton.

Tart, C. (Ed.). (1976). *Transpersonal psychologies*. New York: Harper & Row.

Taylor, R. (1974). *Metaphysics* (2nd ed.). Englewood Cliffs, NJ: Prentice-Hall.

CHAPTER 6

Nature of Human Life as Subject Matter of Nursing

"The most beautiful thing we can experience is the mysterious. It is the source of all true art and science."

—ANONYMOUS

BASIC BELIEFS

My theory of human care begins with my view of personhood and human existence; that in itself becomes metaphysical. What is essential in human existence is that the human has transcended nature—yet remains a part of it. The human can go forward, through the use of the mind, to higher levels of consciousness by finding meaning and harmony in existence.

My conception of life and personhood is tied to notions that one's soul possesses a body that is not confined by objective time and space. The lived world of the experiencing person is not distinguished by external and internal notions of time and space but shapes its own time and space, which is unconstrained by linearity. Notions of personhood, then, transcend the here and now, and one has the capacity to coexist with past, present, and future, all at once. As a result of this view, there is a great deal of regard, respect, and awe given to the concept of a human soul (spirit or higher sense of self) that is greater than the physical, mental, and emotional existence of a person at any given point in time. The individual spirit of a person or of collective humanity may continue to exist throughout time, keeping alive a higher sense of humankind. Although a body may die, be murdered, kill itself, be diseased, be infirmed, and so on, the soul or spirit continues to live on. However, the soul can be underdeveloped, dormant, and in need of reawakening.

According to Jung (1968, p. 99),

> People will do anything, no matter how absurd, in order to avoid facing their own soul. They will practice yoga and all its exercises, observe a strict regime of diet, learn theosophy by heart, or mechanically repeat mystic texts from the literature of the whole world—all because they cannot get on with themselves and have not the slightest faith that anything useful could ever come out of their own soul.

The belief that a person possesses a soul is to be regarded as sacred, to honor with the deepest respect, dignity, mystery, and awe because of the continuing, yet unknown, journey throughout time and space, infinite and external. The soul then exists for something larger, greater, and more powerful than physical life as we know it and could know it for time past, time present, and time future.

The concept of the soul, as used here, refers to the geist, spirit, inner self, or essence of the person, which is connected to higher source of infinity, of the cosmos, and is tied to a greater sense of self-awareness, a higher degree of consciousness, an inner strength, and a power that can expand human capacities and allow a person to transcend his or her usual self. The higher sense of consciousness and valuing of inner self can cultivate a fuller access to the intuitive and even sometimes allow uncanny, mystical, or miraculous experiences, modes of thought, feelings, and actions that we have all experienced at some points in our life but from which our rational, scientific cultures bar us. The terms "soul," "inner self," "spiritual self," and "geist" all refer to the same phenomenon and tend to be used interchangeably.

One's ability to transcend time and space occurs in a similar manner through one's mind, imagination, and emotions. Our bodies may be physically present in a given location or situation, but our minds and related feelings may be located elsewhere.

For example, I have a body but I am not just my body. I have emotions and thoughts, but I am not my emotions and thoughts. We transcend and exist beyond body, emotional, and mental experience; our true self, higher self, transpersonal self is beyond. The transpersonal perspective allows us to go beyond physical-ego self to quiet depths of the soul, beneath the turbulent waves of the passing experiences, and connect with that which is timeless and eternal—the *eternal moment* that Whitehead wrote about (Watson, 2011).

Each of the assumptions underlying the view of human life is that each of us is a magnificent spiritual being who has often been undernourished and reduced to a physical, materialistic being. We know both rationally and intuitively, however, that a person's human predicament may not be related to the external, physical world as much as to the person's inner world as lived and experienced. Awareness of one's self as a spiritual being opens up infinite possibilities.

Poets, sages, and philosophers throughout time have referred to the spiritual side of life and living and have advocated that self-knowledge, self-reverence, self-control, and even self-healing come from the inner, spiritual self, from an inner process that connects one with the life source through the miracle of breathing in spirit and source of life. The notion of a spiritual self and inner power that connect us with a universal source requires a different starting point for how we view people, existence, life, the world, and our universe. The idea of transcendence is fairly alien to the Western world with its mind–body schism. Yet ancient civilizations, philosophers, and poets have long believed, practiced, and written about the transcendence of self, higher consciousness, over-soul, spiritual experience, miracles, mystical experiences, and so on.

The idea of transcendence represents options for true human growth and an evolving human consciousness of our relationship with the infinite field of life itself; it offers opportunities to become more fully human and evolve toward greater spiritual depths. The views inherent in these ideas allow one to turn inward and regard oneself and others with reverence and dignity, as spiritual beings capable of contributing to the spiritual evolution of self and civilization.

LIFE

Human life in this instance, then, is defined as spiritually, mentally, emotionally, and physically being-in-the-world as a unitary being, which is continuous in time and space. Only to the extent that a person has fulfilled the concrete meaning of human existence will the self be fulfilled. The meaning that a being has to fulfill is something beyond the self; it is never just self. The approach herein incorporates scientific views and research with a deep philosophy of the goodness of humankind with a sense of aesthetics and spiritual growth to become more cosmically conscious, adhering to metaphysics.

Because of these values and beliefs about life and personhood, it follows that access to the higher sense of self comes more readily through the human emotions, the mind, and the subjective inner life world of the experiencing person. It also follows from Nightingale forward that healing comes from nature and is an inner process, not an external one.

In developing a theory of nursing, it is helpful to clarify one's values and views of human life because those underlying values and beliefs give direction and meaning to nursing, the human caring process, and other components of the theory. The human caring process between a nurse and another individual is a special, delicate gift to be cherished. The human caring moments and connections provide a coming together and establishment of contact between persons; one's whole being engages with another's whole being in a spirit-to-spirit as well as physical presence in a lived moment. The shared moment of the present has the potential to transcend time and space and the physical, concrete world as we generally view it in the traditional nurse–patient relationship.

Each person (both nurse and patient) brings to the present moment his or her own unique perceptual, experiential and "causal past."* Each experiential moment of "now" becomes incorporated into one's causal past and helps to direct one's future. All three phases of time (past, present, future) can be, and usually are, operating in the inner and lived world of the experiencing person.

---

*This term derives from Whitehead (1967) and involves collective but unique past experiences and events that each person brings to the present moment. Each person's causal past and presentational immediacy have the potential to influence the future.

A person's inner world can transcend time past, present, and future through introspection, creative imagination, meditation, visualization, and the projection of the self in a series of experiences, as well as in sleep, dreaming, and fantasizing, including unconscious and possibly supraconscious processes not yet known or fully explored.

ILLNESS

Illness is not necessarily disease. Illness is subjective turmoil or disharmony within a person's inner self or soul at some level or disharmony with the person. In a situation where one's "I" is separated from one's "me," the self is separated from the self or one's soul. Illness connotes a felt incongruence within the person such as an incongruence between the self as perceived and the self as experienced.

A troubled inner soul can lead to illness, and illness can produce disease. Specific experiences, for example, developmental conflicts, inner suffering, guilt, self-blame, despair, loss, and grief, and general and specific stress can lead to illness and result in disease. Unknowns can also lead to illness; the unknown can only be known by experience and may require inner searching to find meaning. Disease processes can also result from genetic, constitutional vulnerabilities and manifest themselves when disharmony is present. Disease itself in turn creates more disharmony.

In this view of illness one may be cured of disease or illness but not be healed; healing is an inner process and has been defined as being-in right-relation by colleague Janet Quinn. Likewise, in this way of considering person, health, illness, and life, a person may not be cured but healed through experiencing the dying process, which facilitated the person being in right relation with dying as ultimate healing.

HEALTH

Health is a subjective experience; it can refer to unity and harmony with body-mind-spirit. Health is also associated with the degree of congruence between the self as perceived and the self as experienced.

Such a view of health focuses on the entire nature of the individual in his or her physical, social, aesthetic, and moral realms—instead of just certain aspects of human behavior and physiology. Such a view is referred to as eudemonistic model of health (Smith, 1983).

In summary,

I = Me—Health (harmony, 'in right-relation,' with self-world and open to increased diversity)

I ≠[does not equal] Me—Illness (in varying degrees and person less open to increased diversity)

When I ≠ me for continuous periods of time, disease may be present.

GOAL

The goal of nursing is to help persons gain a higher degree of harmony that fosters self-knowledge, self-reverence, self-caring, self-control, and self-healing processes while allowing increasing diversity. This goal is pursued through the human-to-human caring process and spirit-to-spirit caring connections and relationship that respond to the subjective inner world of the person in such a way that the nurse helps individuals find meaning in their existence, disharmony, suffering, and turmoil and promotes self-control, choice, self-knowledge and informed self-determination with health–illness decisions.

Nursing contributes to the human caring sciences by establishing a set of values, assumptions, ethics, philosophical orientation, goals, and methods about humans and science that seek to integrate and unify:

- The unity of human mind-body-soul as inseparable one whole (as contrasted to a particulate view of the body)
- Reality and fantasy
- Facts and meaning
- Objective and subjective worlds
- External and internal events
- Disease, illness, and health
- Physical and metaphysical realms

Society needs the caring professions, and nursing in particular, to help to restore humanity and nourish the human heart and soul in an age of technology, scientism, loneliness, rapid change, and stresses, an age without moral or ethical wisdom, as to how to serve humanity.

This particular theory of nursing is metaphysical in that it goes beyond the rapidly emerging existential–phenomenological approaches in nursing (for example, Paterson, Zderad, Parse, Taddy, and the important approaches of Rogers, Newman, King, and others) to a higher level of abstraction and a higher sense of personhood, which incorporates the concept of the soul and transcendence. The notion of a human soul is nothing new or original. It is, however, unusual to include it in a theory. The closest concept in psychology and nursing are concepts like self, inner self, I, me, self-actualization, and so on. The bold attempt to acknowledge and incorporate a concept of the soul in a nursing theory is a reflection of an alternative position that nursing is now free to take. This new concept breaks from the traditional medical science model and is also a reflection of the scientific times. The evolution of the history and philosophy of science now allows some attention to metaphysical views that would have been unacceptable at an earlier point in time.

My basic beliefs and values about human life provide a foundation for my theory of nursing and become an integral part of nursing goals and nursing human caring connections and relations. They also influence the subject matter of the theory, the perspective on the subject matter, and the approach for reasoning and for "seeing" the human-universe phenomenon in front of us.

Basic Premise

1. A person's consciousness and emotions are windows to the soul. Nursing care can be and is physical, procedural, objective, and factual, but at the highest level of nursing the nurses' human caring responses, the human caring connections and the nurses' presence in the relationship transcend the physical and material world, bound in time and space, and make contact with the person's spirit-filled subjective world as the route to the inner self and the higher sense of self. So we open to an evolving consciousness throughout the lifetime to evolve toward a higher consciousness. We may pose the question, What is the highest level of consciousness? Is it not love? Are we not evolving to become more loving, and therefore more godly, as God is love?

2. A person's body is confined in time and space, but the mind and soul are not confined to the physical universe. One's higher sense of mind and soul transcends time and space and helps to account for notions like collective unconsciousness, causal past, mystical experiences, parapsychological phenomena, miracles, and a higher sense of power and may be an indicator of the spiritual evolution of human beings. (This idea has been proposed by numerous philosophers, including Teilhard de Chardin, Kierkegaard, Hegel, and Marcel.) De Chardin (1967) indicated that humans are evolving toward an "omega point" to become more holy, more God-conscious.

3. A nurse may have access to a person's mind, emotions, and inner self indirectly through any sphere—mind, body, or soul—provided the physical body is not perceived or treated as separate from the mind and emotions

and higher sense of self (soul). This is consistent with Hippocrates, who thought the person's mind and soul should be inspired before illness could be treated.

4. The spirit, inner self, or soul (geist) of a person exists in and for itself. The spiritual essence of the person is related to the human ability to be free, which is an evolving process in the development of humans. The ability to develop and experience one's essence freely is limited by the extent of others' ability to "be." The destiny of one's being (humankind's destiny) is to develop the spiritual essence of the self and, in the highest sense, to become more god-like. One person's level of humanity is reflected onto others and each of us. Therefore, each person has to question his or her own essence and moral behavior toward others, because if people are dehumanized at a basic level, for example, a human caring level, that dehumanizing process is not capable of reflecting humanity back upon itself; it is reflecting dehumanizing, objectification, reducing other to moral status of object, allowing us to do things to other as object we would not do to a whole person.

5. People need each other in a caring, loving way. Love and caring are two universal givens. To paraphrase Teilhard de Chardin, Love (and care) are the most universal, the most tremendous, and the most mysterious of cosmic forces. . . It is the primal and universal psychic energy (1967). These needs are often overlooked, because even though we know we need one another in a loving and caring way, we do not behave well toward each other. If our humanness is to survive, we need to become more loving, caring, and moral to nourish our humanity, advance as a civilization, and live together. As a beginning we have to impose our own will to love, care, and be moral upon our own behavior, not on others' behavior. We need to love, respect, and care for ourselves and treat ourselves with dignity before we can respect, love, and care for others and treat them with dignity.

6. A person may have an illness or even disease that is completely hidden from our eyes. To find solutions it is necessary to find meanings. A person's human predicament may not be related to the external world as much as to the person's inner world as he or she experiences it.

7. The totality of experience at any given moment constitutes an energetic, phenomenal life field. The energetic, phenomenal field is the individual's frame of reference and comprises the subjective internal relations and the meanings of objects, subjects, past, present, and future as perceived and experienced. This energetic field is connected to the universal life source field of infinity.

A PERSONAL ANECDOTAL NOTE FOR STUDENTS

Rose McKay, an earlier nursing historian, educator, and scholar, suggested to me that the ideas represented by these values, goals, and beliefs lead to a prescriptive theory for nursing. That is, if nursing assumes it now has the professional disciplinary development, assumes it has a knowledge base and can assume competency, these ideas suggest we are now ready to review what we do with our knowledge, professional maturity and competencies. As such they suggest a moral ideal and moral commitment.

These notions were posed to me in the spring of 1982 by Professor Rose McKay in her graduate theory class. The other issue raised by Dr. McKay was the overlap in my ideas between a philosophy and a theory. I am quite sure my ideas represent some of both but not either exclusively.

In viewing my ideas as helping nursing and nurses to develop a meaningful philosophical base for one's practice and our science and to examine what we stand for scientifically, socially, and morally, these do call for renewal and rededication in an age of professional confusion. I do not think of myself as having a prescriptive theory, and I even question whether nursing can truly have a prescriptive theory. Perhaps, however, the human values and moral ideals are foundationally prescriptive. These rhetorical ideas and unanswered questions can serve as teaching guides for students to critique and debate as part of the evolving discourse of nursing theory.

REFERENCES

de Chardin, T. (1967). *On love* (pp. 7–8). New York: Harper & Row.

Jung, C. G. (1968). Psychology and alchemy. In H. Read, M. Fordham, & G. Adler (Eds.), *The collected works of C.G. Jung* (vol. 12, pp. 99–101). Princeton, NJ: Princeton University Press.

Quinn, J. F. (1992). Holding sacred space: The nurse as healing environment. *Holistic Nursing Practice*, 6(4), 26–35.

Smith, J. (1983). *The idea of health* (p. 31). New York: Teachers College.

Watson, J. (2011). *Postmodern nursing and beyond* (p. 167). Boulder, CO: Watson Caring Science Institute.

Whitehead, A. N. (1967) *Science and the modern world.* New York: The Free Press.

BIBLIOGRAPHY

de Chardin, T. (1967). *On love.* New York: Harper & Row.

Jung, C. G. (1968). Psychology and alchemy. In H. Read, M. Fordham, & G. Adler (Eds.), *The collected works of C.G. Jung* (vol. 12). Princeton, NJ: Princeton University Press.

Smith, J. (1983). *The idea of health.* New York: Teachers College.

CHAPTER 7

Theory Components
and Definitions

*"The human mind is forever moving. The activities of the mind have
no limit, they form the surroundings of life. Surroundings have no
more limits than the activities of the mind."*

—Baddyo Dendo Kyakai, *The Teachings of Buddha**

This chapter is an extension of Chapter 6 and includes more components of
the theory, definitions of specific terms, and how they interrelate.

DEFINITION OF NURSING

The word nursing is a philosophical concept that suggests tenderness and
holds various meanings for people. As such, the concept of nursing is dynamic
and changing. The word "nurse" is both a noun and a verb. "Nursing" also stands
as a metaphor for caring–healing, wholeness, and connection with inner processes
and yin energy to access sacred nature of human experiences and greater source
for healing, beyond treating the body physical alone. As Nightingale (1859)
reminds us: The care of the body can never be separate from care of the soul.

There are many facets to nursing and the meaning of nurse. There is the
nurse as a person and the nurse who holds a caring-loving consciousness and
intentionality toward self and other that is manifest in specific responses, behaviors, and informed actions. Nursing to me generally consists of knowledge,
thought, values, philosophy, commitment, and action, with some degree of passion. The knowledge, values, action, and passion are generally related to human
caring moments and to intersubjective, personal, human-to-human contact with
the lived world of the experiencing person.

As such, human care/caring is viewed as the moral ideal of nursing. It consists of transpersonal human-to-human attempts to protect, enhance, and preserve humanity and human dignity, integrity and wholeness, by helping a person
find meaning in illness, suffering, pain, and existence and to help another gain
self-knowledge, self-control, self-caring, and self-healing wherein a sense of
inner harmony is restored regardless of the external circumstances. The nurse

---

The Teachings of Buddha (4th ed.). Tokyo: Kosaido Printing Co. Ltd., 1976.

helps the person "be-in-right-relation" with self/other and the wider universe (Quinn, personal communication and definition of healing).

The nurse is a coparticipant in a process in which the ideal of caring is intersubjectivity and human-to-human connections. Because of the human nature of nursing, the moral, spiritual, and metaphysical components of nursing cannot be ignored or replaced. They are inherently operating, directly or indirectly, and therefore need to be acknowledged as part of a theorist's world view, belief system, and philosophy. In a sense, the metaphysical beliefs of a nursing theory provide the passion for nursing and keep it alive, changing, and open to increasing diversity and new possibilities.

SCIENCE AND DISCIPLINE OF NURSING

Nursing in this context may be defined as a human caring science of persons and human health–illness experiences that are mediated by professional, personal, scientific, aesthetic, and ethical human care connections and relationships. Such a view requires the nurse to be a scientist, scholar, and clinician but also a humanitarian and moral agent, wherein the nurse as a person is engaged as an active coparticipant in the human caring process and relationships. This human caring science orientation leans toward using qualitative theories and research methods, such as existential–phenomenology, literary introspection, case studies, philosophical–historical/work, narrative, stories, artistic expressions, and even performance as a contemporary form of inquiry and research. Other approaches will continue to evolve that allow a close and systematic observation of one's own and other's human experiences and inner subjective processes that seek to disclose and elucidate the lived world of human health–illness experience and the phenomena of human-to-human caring and healing.

Because nursing science involves intersubjective relational human-to-human caring, the process and practice of nursing become transpersonal and metaphysical. When these aspects of nursing are acknowledged and incorporated into our science, nursing can cultivate a fuller access of the intuitive, aesthetic, quasi-rational modes of thought, feeling, and action, and there can be greater use of our geist or spirit in relating to others from which the rational, Western scientific culture often closes off.

This position does not discount scientific method or Western thought; rather, it seeks to elucidate and acknowledge the other dimensions operating, if we are to understand the idea of the person, nursing, and human caring–healing processes in health and illness.

The person is viewed as "a spiritual being-in-the-world" and is the locus of human existence. The person exists as a living, growing gestalt. The person is viewed as whole and complete with unity of mind-body-spirit. The mind, consciousness, and emotions are the starting point, the focal point, and the point of access to the body and soul. The person is not simply an organism or material physical being; the person is also connected with nature and a spiritual being, neither purely physical nor purely spiritual. A person's existence is embodied in experience, in nature, and in the physical world, but a person can also transcend the physical world and nature by influencing it, changing it, repatterning it, or living in harmony with it.

A person is the experiencing and perceiving spiritual being. As viewed by Teihard de Chardin, the human is a spiritual being having a physical experience on the earth plane. "The self is a fluid and changing gestalt, a process, but at any moment a specific entity" (Rogers, 1959, p. 200).

One's self is a process, an unending process wherein new experience is turned into knowledge and each experiential moment shapes the next experiential moment. In addition to the self as it is, there is an ideal self the person would like to be. The highest sense of the self connotes the spiritual self, the geist, soul, or the essence of the person's self with the "potential forms of consciousness entirely different from our waking consciousness" (James, 1950, p. 305).

The totality of human experience (one's being-in-the-world) constitutes a phenomenal field.[†] The phenomenal field is the individual's frame of reference that can be known only to the person. "It can never be known to another except through empathetic inference and then can never be perfectly known" (Rogers, 1959, p. 210). How a person perceives and responds in a given situation depends on the phenomenal field (subjective reality) and not just on the objective conditions or external reality.

A continuity of consciousness occurs over time. Each successive moment of awareness is shaped by the previous moment and determines the following moment. "The human is like a river that keeps a constant form, though not a single drop is the same as a moment ago" (Van Aung, 1972, p. 7). A person's mental and emotional state and phenomenal field may vary from moment to moment as well as his or her sensory objects—sounds, smells, taste, sights, random memories, and future plans. Other thoughts mingle with and are often associated with objects of the senses and become part of the phenomenal field.

The phenomenal field is not identical with the consciousness but incorporates consciousness along with perceptions of self and others: Feelings, thoughts, bodily sensations, spiritual beliefs, desires, goals, and expectations; environmental considerations; and meanings and the symbolic nature of one's perceptions—all this is based on one's collective consciousness, life history, and the presenting moment as well as the imaged or envisioned future.

[†]These ideas are influenced by writings on gestalt psychology and existential psychology by Carl Rogers, Kurt Goldstein, and Kurt Lewin, as well as by Eastern psychology.

SPIRITUAL DIMENSION

The world of the spirit and soul becomes increasingly more important as a person grows and matures as an individual and as humankind evolves collectively. The salience of the spiritual aspect of a person or race varies from individual to individual, from culture to culture, and within them. As William James (1950, p. 305) said, "Our normal waking consciousness is but one special type of consciousness, whilst all about it, parted from it by the filmiest of screens, there lie potential forms of consciousness entirely different."

Some cultures can be considered more spiritually evolved than others. For example, the Eastern cultures of India and Egypt and countries such as Thailand, Brazil, and other ancient indigenous cultures, with their long histories of spiritual valuing and connectedness with the spirit work and nature, can be viewed as more spiritually developed and having a greater capacity for higher levels of consciousness than our Anglo-Saxon, Western world, with its values on physical materialism combined with the Western world's relatively short history. There is evidence, however, that the Western world's values are moving toward integration of Eastern philosophical views and expanded spiritualism. This movement is manifest in the increase of Eastern philosophies and ideas that are incorporated into health programs, yoga, exercise, health foods, fasting, meditation, and special diets. The works of Gardner Murphy and Lois Murphy in Asian psychology reported quite a number of years ago that the psychological interests of the East and West are quickly coming together (Murphy & Murphy, 1968).

The world refers to all these dimensions of a unitary world view and evolving universe as well as to a person's immediate environment and situation that affect the person. These dimensions may be internal, external, human, artificial, natural, cosmic, psychic, infinite, past, present, or future.

Harmony–Disharmony

Where there is disharmony among the mind, body, and soul or between a person and his or her nature and relationship with a larger world/universe, there is a disjunctive between the self as perceived and one's actual experience. There is also a perceived incongruence within the person, between the I and me, and between the person and the world. Incongruence between the self as perceived and a person's experience reflects the presence of disharmony within the soul and seems disconnected from the person—the I is not equal to the real self or the real me. This incongruence leads to threat, anxiety, and inner turmoil and can lead to a sense of existential despair, dread, and illness. If prolonged, it can contribute to disease.

If there is harmony and unity of mind-body-spirit, then a sense of congruence exists between the I and me; between the self as perceived and the self as experienced by the person: a felt sense of being-in-right-relation.

Another element of congruence–incongruence is the congruence—or lack of it—between subjective reality (the phenomenal field) and external reality (the world as it is). If a person does not feel in-right-relation, he or she may reject self or be obsessed with or even reject the higher self, leading to dissatisfaction and lack of self-love and self-acceptance. Thus, this incongruence can result in a lack of union with another human or cause a person to feel separate, disconnected, and alone in his or her quest to be-in-right-relation and grow. Another type of incongruence can occur if there is a lack of harmony between a person and nature; such a position calls attention to the need for the human to live in harmony with nature and aesthetics in one's world. There is increasing evidence of the relationship between human caring and eco-caring if the Earth and humans are to survive into the future.

Striving

The person has one basic struggle: to actualize the real self, thereby developing the spiritual essence of the self, and in the highest sense to become more god-like. Goethe reminded us that human striving is a quality of life; it is evolutionary and offers a beautiful purpose to our existence. It is the basis of human experience of persistence, to keep going with both the good and the bad in life and life's journey. We learn that we may control our start of things but must learn to let go of the end point, that we are not fully in control and must learn to "let things happen" in spite of our striving, desire, and need to evolve to become more spirit filled, more connected with our divinity.

Each person seeks harmony, integrity, and unity with self in relation to others, community, environment, nature, the universe, and the source. The more one is able to experience one's self in right-relation with the source, the more harmony there will be, and a higher degree of health/wholeness will exist. Because disharmony is associated with illness and harmony is associated with health, the nursing profession is concerned with how disharmony develops and how the self can be helped to be in right-relation with the source. The nurse caring relationship and human-to-human connection contribute to the person's developing spiritual essence. The nurse seeks to "see" who is that spirit-filled person, behind the disease, the diagnosis, even the behavior we may not like. Thus, honoring the whole person helps to promote more self-knowledge, self-reverence, self-caring, self-control, and self-healing for both nurse and patient.

Human behavior is basically the goal-directed attempt of the person to satisfy needs as experienced in the perceived phenomenal field. Although there are many needs, each of them is subservient to basic striving toward actualizing one's spiritual self and establishing harmony and right-relation with the source.

In early life the person is more attentive to a sense of harmony between mind/emotions and body. However, as one grows and allows for the existential and spiritual side of one's self to develop, the person becomes more concerned with incongruence or disharmony within if not in right-relation with the soul and the source.

As a person matures he or she becomes more differentiated and his or her sense of inner self becomes more developed. The person then seeks a greater degree of harmony with his or her soul because of a higher sense of discrimination.

Human needs consist of the need to be loved and cared for and about, the need for positive regard, and the need to be accepted, understood, appreciated, and valued (Watson, 1979). There is also a human need to achieve union, transcend one's individual life, and find harmony with life.

TRANSPERSONAL CARING MOMENT

Transpersonal human care and human caring relationships are those scientific, professional, and ethical, yet aesthetic, creative, and personalized life-giving–life-receiving behaviors and responses between two people (nurse and other) that allow for contact between the subjective world of the experiencing persons (through physical, mental, or spiritual routes or some combination thereof).‡ The transpersonal human caring moments and connections include the nurse's consciousness, intentionality, and unique energetic healing presence, through full use of self through movements, senses, touch, sounds, words, colors, and forms in which he or she transmits and reflects the person's condition back to that person. He or she does this in such a way that allows for the release and flow of his or her intersubjective feelings and thoughts and pent-up energy. This transpersonal caring moment can be transcendent in that it opens up shared access to a spirit-filled source of infinity. Such caring connections in turn help to restore inner harmony while also contributing to the

---

‡Transpersonal refers to an intersubjective, transcendent, human-to-human relationship in which the person of the nurse affects and is affected by the person of the other. Both are fully present in the moment and feel a union with the other. They share a phenomenal field that becomes part of the life history of both, and they are coparticipants in becoming in the now and the future. Such an ideal of caring entails an ideal of intersubjectivity, in which both persons are involved. The human transpersonal spirit-to-spirit connection opens up shared access to the source, the mystery, and the infinite unitary field of the universe—that which connects us with the sacred circle of life.

patient and nurse finding meaning in the experience. However, the origin of the meaning for both resides within rather than existing without. In this process the nurse is also attending to a concern above all for the dignity of the person as an important end. Dignity in this sense "simply expressed as being has dignity when it gives to itself, its meaning and so creates for itself integrity" (Gadow, 1984, p. 6).

The contact with the subjective world has the potential to go beyond bodily or mental–emotional contact or interaction and to reach out and touch the higher, spiritual sense of self or the soul. As such, transpersonal human caring occurs from person to person in an I–Thou relationship. It can release inner power and strength and help the person gain a sense of inner harmony. This contact and process in turn generates and potentiates the self-healing processes.

The two individuals (nurse and other) in a transpersonal caring moment are both in a process of being and becoming. Both individuals bring with them to the relationship a unique life history and phenomenal field, and both are influenced and affected by the nature of the relationship and connection, which in turn becomes part of the life history of each person. In this sense of a caring moment, caring is a moral ideal rather than an interpersonal technique, and it entails a commitment to a particular end. The end is the protection, enhancement, and preservation of the person's humanity and human dignity, which helps to restore inner harmony, wholeness, and potential healing.

An Actual Caring Moment Occasion

Two persons (nurse and other) together with their unique life histories and phenomenal field in a human caring connection comprise an event.[§] An event, such as an actual occasion of human caring, is a focal point in time and space from which experience and perception are taking place, but the actual moment of caring has a field of its own that is greater than the occasion itself. As such, the process can go beyond itself yet arise from aspects of itself that become part of the life history of each person as well as part of some larger, deeper, complex pattern of life (Figure 7-1).

An actual caring moment occasion involves action and choice both by the nurse and the individual. The moment of coming together in a caring moment occasion presents the two persons with the opportunity to decide how to be in the relationship—what to do with the moment. Whatever is decided involves one manner and not another. If the caring moment occasion is indeed transpersonal and allows for the presence of the geist or spirit of both, then the moment

---

[§]Based on Whitehead's notion of EVENT, the actual occasion (Whitehead, 1953).

Figure 7-1   Transpersonal caring moment.

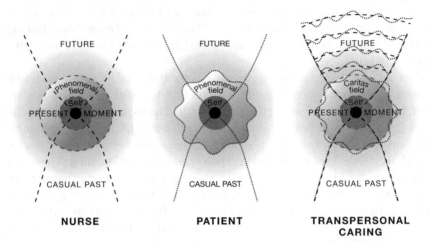

expands the limits of openness and has the ability to expand the human capacities. It thereby increases the range of certain events that could occur in time and space at that moment as well as in the future. The occasion of the caring moment becomes part of the past life history of both persons and presents both with new opportunities.

Such an ideal of intersubjectivity and spirit-to-spirit connection between the nurse and patient is based on a belief that we learn from one another how to be human by identifying ourselves with others or finding their dilemmas in ourselves. What we all learn from it is self-knowledge. The self we learn about or discover is every self: It is universal—the human self. We learn to recognize ourselves in others. The comparison shows us what we are, what humanness is in general, and, in particular, the intersubjectivity keeps alive our common humanity and avoids reducing the human being to an object.

A transpersonal human caring and in a caring moment, the nurse can enter into the experience of another person and another can enter into the nurse's experience. The ideal of transpersonal caring is an ideal of intersubjectivity in which both persons are involved. This means that the value and views of the nurse, although not decisive, are potentially as relevant as those of the patient. A refusal to allow the nurse's subjectivity to be engaged by a patient is, in effect, a refusal to recognize the validity of the patient's subjectivity. The alternative to caring as intersubjectivity is not simply the reduction of the patient to the moral status of an object, but the reduction of the nurse to that level as well (Gadow, 1984).

When including the metaphysical components of the spiritual experience in the intersubjective caring moment, the nurse is allowed to experience and explain things yet does not have to concern him- or herself with full prediction. He or she is able, however, to include the mysteries of life and unknowns yet to be discovered.

A transpersonal caring moment is located not only in the simple physical instance of a given moment of time, but the event/experience has internal relations to other objects-subjects in the phenomenal field plus internal subjective relations between the past, present, and imagined future for each person and for the whole. An actual caring moment can be present in the life of both the nurse and person beyond the physical instance of the given point in time. Thus, a caring moment transcends time, space, and physicality. Each moment informs the next moment and affects the life of each person.

Time

One cannot clearly distinguish between past and present time even though the present is more subjectively real and the past is both objectively and subjectively real. The past is prior to or in a different mode of being than the present, but it is not clearly distinguishable. Past, present, and future instants merge and fuse. Whitehead (1953) uses the notion of "the eternal now" to capture the experience that past/present/future are contained in a given moment in time.

The notion of the caring moment and transcendence of time is depicted by Virginia Woolf in "A Writer's Diary" (1975, p. 374):

> Friday, January 4th. "Now is life very solid or very shifting? I am haunted by the two contradictions. This has gone on forever; will last forever; goes down to the bottom of the world—this moment I stand on. Also it is transitory, flying, diaphanous. I shall pass like a cloud on the waves. Perhaps it may be that though we change, one flying after another, so quick, so quick, yet we are somehow successive and continuous we human beings; and show the light through."

Figure 7-1 depicts the various components of transpersonal caring, including self, phenomenal field, and actual caring moment/occasion of the patient and nurse, intersubjectively coming together in a given moment in time whereby the past, present, and future merge. The actual caring moment in a presenting instant has the potential to influence both nurse and patient in the future. The caring moment and this presenting occasion then become part of the subjective, lived reality and the life history of both. Both are coparticipants in becoming in the now and the future, and both are part of some larger, deeper, complex pattern of life.

REFERENCES

de Chardin, T. (1967). *On love* (pp. 7–8). New York: Harper & Row.

Gadow, S. (1984). Existential advocacy as a form of caring: Technology, truth, and touch. Paper presented to the Research Seminar Series: The Development of Nursing as a Human Science. The School of Nursing, University of Colorado Health Sciences Center. Denver, March.

James, W. (1950). *The principles of psychology*. New York: Dover.

Murphy, G., & Murphy, L. B. (Eds.). (1968). *Asian psychology*. New York: Basic Books.

Nightingale, F. (1959). *Notes on Nursing*. London: Harrison.

Rogers, C. R. (1959). A theory of therapy, personality, and interpersonal relationships, as developed in the client-centered framework. In S. Koch (Ed.), *Psychology: A study of a science* (vol. 3). New York: McGraw-Hill.

Van Aung, Z. (Ed. and Trans.). (1972). *Compendium of philosophy*. London: Pali Text Society.

Watson, J. (1979). *Nursing: The philosophy and science of caring* (pp. 183–193). Boston: Little, Brown.

Whitehead, A. N. (1953). *Science and the modern world*. Cambridge, UK: Cambridge University Press.

Woolf, V. (1975). A writer's diary. In J. Hersey (Ed.), *The writer's craft* (p. 374). New York: Knopf.

BIBLIOGRAPHY

Gadow, S. (1984). Existential advocacy as a form of caring: Technology, truth, and touch. Paper presented to the Research Seminar Series: The Development of Nursing as a Human Science. The School of Nursing, University of Colorado Health Sciences Center, Denver, March.

Guenther, H.V. (1976). *Philosophy and psychology in the abhidhamma*. Berkeley, CA: Shambhala.

James, W. (1950). *The principles of psychology*. New York: Dover.

Murphy, G., & Murphy, L. B. (Eds.). (1968). *Asian psychology*. New York: Basic Books.

Rogers, C. R. (1959). A theory of therapy, personality, and interpersonal relationships, as developed in the client-centered framework. In S. Koch (Ed.), *Psychology: A study of a science* (vol. 3). New York: McGraw-Hill.

Van Aung, Z. (Ed. and Trans.). (1972). *Compendium of philosophy*. London: Palli Text Society.

Watson, J. (1979). *Nursing: The philosophy and science of caring*. Boston: Little, Brown.

Whitehead, A. N. (1953). *Science and the modern world*. Cambridge, UK: Cambridge University Press.

Woolf, V. (1975). A writer's diary. In J. Hersey (Ed.), *The writer's craft* (p. 374). New York: Knopf.

CHAPTER 8

Transpersonal Caring Relationship

A transpersonal caring relationship connotes a special kind of human care relationship—a connection/union with another person, a high regard for the whole person and their being-in-the-world. Caring, in this sense, is viewed as the moral ideal of nursing where there is the utmost concern for human dignity and preservation of humanity. Human caring begins when the nurse enters into the life space or phenomenal field of another person, is able to detect the other person's condition of being (spirit, soul), feels this condition within him- or herself, and responds to the condition in such a way that the recipient has a release of subjective feelings and thoughts he or she had been longing to release. As such, there is an intersubjective flow between the nurse and patient. As feelings, thoughts, and energies that are less harmonious with either person's self are released, they become replaced by other feelings, thoughts, and energies that are more harmonious with one's self and are kinder toward and more mindful of the well-being of each person and ultimately for humankind.

The simple, yet complex, human-to-human caring process in nursing is a very basic foundation and starting point from which a harmonizing transpersonal caring relationship can occur. The nurse enters into the space with the other, and from a 'centered' ground of intentional presence, pauses and seeks 'to see' who is that spirit-filled person behind the patient; behind the disease; behind the diagnosis; even behind the behavior one may not condone or approve. The nurse's very heart-centered caring presence and conscious intentionality creates open space where something new can happen, greater than what may have been assumed. In this complex but compassionate being and connecting, the nurse is helping to put the patient in the best condition to access his or her own inner healing resources, connecting with a universal source for healing and renewal, even allowing for miracles. (By miracles, I mean allowing and opening to something happening that is beyond expectations and beyond normal occurrences one may anticipate). This process is congruent with Nightingale's model of putting the patient in the best condition for nature to heal.

A transpersonal caring relationship depends on several factors:

1. A moral commitment to protect and enhance human dignity, wherein a person is allowed to determine his or her own meaning.
2. The nurse's intent and will to affirm the subjective, spiritual significance of the person (I–Thou honoring relationship of mutuality versus I–It relationship).
3. The nurse's ability to realize and accurately detect feelings and the inner condition of another. To seek 'to see' and connect spirit-to-spirit with the other, even in the moment. This can occur through authentic presence, being open, intentional and mindful with actions, words, behaviors, cognition, body language, feelings, thought, senses, intuition, and so on.
4. The ability of the nurse to assess and realize another's condition of being-in-the-world and to feel a human-to-human connection with another. The nurse must be able to express the condition and/or attend to the condition through various means, such as movement, gestures, looks, acts, procedures, information, touch, sound, words, color, and form and other similar scientific, aesthetic, and human means. The subjectivity of the patient is assumed to be as whole and as valid as that of the nurse. Mutuality, therefore, is a moral foundation of nursing. (If conditions 1 through 4 are present, the one being cared for is better able to have a release of some of his or her inner disharmony and to be more free to authentically express and directly release his or her true heart-felt feelings and needs; his or her pent-up energy, accessing his or her own healing process.)
5. The nurse's own life history (collective past) and previous experiences, culture, background, and opportunities of having lived through or experienced one's own feelings and various human conditions and of having imagined others' feelings and sufferings from various human conditions. Such knowledge and sensitivity can be gained through working with other cultures; the study of the humanities, art, drama, and literature; exploring values; exploring one's relationship with self; cultivating loving kindness and equanimity with self; and honoring one's self caring compassionate relationship with self. It can also be facilitated through values clarification, personal psychotherapy, meditation, prayer, journaling, self-healing practices, yoga, Shamanic experiences, nature, practice of silence, inner journeying, and so on. It is related to personal growth, maturity, the evolution of the person's consciousness and spiritual awareness and practices, and development of the nurse's self, sensitivity to self and others, and a deeply human-universe value system.

USE OF ENTIRE SELF IN NURSING

The introduction of the professional nurse as a person in a transpersonal relationship with the patient may conflict with traditional views of the professional nurse. Nurses and other health professionals have been warned to avoid personal interactions, and personal involvement is considered unprofessional. Sally Gadow (1980) makes a convincing case for softening the distinction between the person and the professional. Her ideas are consistent with a transpersonal caring moment and human caring spirit-to-spirit connections and the notion of *transpersonal,* which implies going-beyond ego-self and connecting with something greater.

Gadow emphasizes that even if responding person to person there will still be important differences between the nurse and patient, although it is still possible to allow the "amount" of the personal involvement to be equal. The concept of professional involvement as the participation of the entire self, using every dimension of the person—all of one's unique gifts, talents, skills, knowledge, intuitions, tastes, perceptions, personality, and so on—as a resource in the professional relationship is entailed in the concept of a transpersonal caring relationship between the nurse and patient. Some personal differences have been classified in terms of (1) focus, (2) intensity, and (3) perspective (Gadow, 1980).

The focus of a patient's personal involvement in a professional relationship, for example, is directed toward the presenting person/situation at hand and its effect on his or her life. The concern is unavoidably self-directed. In contrast, the personal involvement of the nurse/person is directed away from one's own (ego) self toward the other's spirit-filled self. The nurse's feelings may be experienced and felt, not as a way of obtaining relief or help from patients but as part of being and becoming and connecting in the relationship, in the moment.

Personal relationships between friends have a give and take process of exchange wherein the one who needs the most receives from the other. However, there is a reciprocal sharing and an accepted norm of mutuality where each party in the relationship helps the other. A professional relationship may indeed benefit the nurse and does allow for the nurse to benefit and be influenced by the other; indeed, the patient may be a messenger of meaning and healing to the nurse, unknowingly; however, the nurse does not depend on receiving from the patient to maintain the involvement.

The intensity of the relationship that Gadow outlines is also experienced differently by the nurse and the patient. The patient experiences the immediacy of the distress. Intensity and, likewise, immediacy may indeed be felt by the nurse, but they serve to generate the reflective process necessary for caring and help to be given. "Being able to help, to hold the other person's pain, suffering and tears, for example, has greater value than simply sharing the other's experience. . . . This is in order to integrate feelings and knowledge in the attempt to alleviate the patient's distress" (Gadow, 1980, pp. 88–89).

Finally, the perspectives of the two persons (nurse and patient) differ. The nurse is externally involved, whereas the patient feels the pain from the inside and knows that it is his or her whole personhood that is affected. There is a felt sense of aloneness, of separation from true self or one's inner heart and soul knowing—of not being-in right-relation with Source.

As Gadow goes on to explain, the difference in perspectives between the two is often used to indicate degrees of emotional involvement. The implication is that the patient is more emotional and the nurse less emotional. There is the real possibility, however, that both persons might (and do) experience emotional intensity.

The professional nurse differs from the patient or a friend in that the nurse helps integrate the subjective experience and emotions with the objective, external view of the situation. Even acknowledging some differences between personal and professional relations, most assumed conditions related to unequal involvement do not exist. For example, the nurse does not manifest less involvement as a person than does the patient. The form and direction of the involvement may differ, but the amount of the nurse's involvement is equally as great. Personal involvement in a professional capacity is not an alternative to other kinds of involvement. It is a synthesis of involvements, a participation of the entire creative self, using every dimension of the person as a resource in the professional relation.

Because nursing is so immediate, and often intimate and private, with scientific, artistic, humanistic, ethical, and technical complexities, it offers avenues for every dimension of the professional including the technical, emotional, mental, aesthetic, intuitive, creative, physical, spiritual, and experiential—to be involved. Thus, an expanded epistemology is acknowledged, honored, and processed as part of the human caring–healing experience that is shared.

At many points throughout life, people are confronted with existential/spiritual concerns about their existence and the meaning of their lives. These concerns tend to be more urgent when the person's existence is threatened. This can occur from a threat to an aspect of one's being, physically, mentally, or spiritually. Indeed, a threat to any one of these aspects of a person in turn affects the others. Decisions are made about one's existence by questioning how one lives one's life, one's relationship with self, and one's priorities, forms of coping, self-caring behaviors, different health and medical practices, degree of help or freedom desired, and so forth.

When the question of meaning arises, people can generally benefit by determining the meaning of their experience. Ideally, a person should have the opportunity for self-determination of the meaning of a health–illness experience before professionals make decisions about treatment or intervention. Indeed, I have heard it said in some contemporary medical circles, that medicine in the future will be less concerned with diagnosis and more concerned with meaning. The meaning one holds in relation to the presenting situation will affect the outcome.

Because the patient has opinions and meanings attached to the health–illness experience the nurse can facilitate free exploration of the meaning and have that meaning incorporated into the person's and the professional's response to the situation. Nursing's continuity with persons often enables the nurse "to experience individuals as unique human beings continuously engaged in creating their own histories" (Gadow, 1980, p. 98). It is when nurses are able to authentically listen to another's story, to hold their suffering for and with them, that may be the greatest healing gift. It is the nurse in that moment who may be the only one who is there to listen to and hold the other's story so he or she can explore their own meaning and thus own self-directed options. It is in this sense of the nurse–patient transpersonal caring relationship that nursing meets the conditions for authentic caring–healing referenced earlier.

At some core level the conflict in nursing in studying and developing ideas of human caring is related to the question of materialism versus spiritualism. The theory of nursing and transpersonal caring is based on the premise that nursing needs "to develop a scientific tradition related to the vast uncharted (by science) sea of human potentials we call spiritual potentialities" (Tart, 1976, p. 58).

The perspective, values, and subject matter developed herein are one attempt to acknowledge and actualize the personal and individual spiritual potentials that can expand through a transpersonal caring relationship. This pursuit is congruent with the theories set forth by Nightingale, who was very clear that nursing is a spiritual practice. When the natural self of the nurse and patient coparticipate in a caring moment, it potentiates self-healing, being-in-right-relation, and human integrity, and there is greater harmony for both nurse and person.

In a transpersonal caring relationship, a spiritual union occurs between the two persons, in which both are capable of transcending self, time, space, and the life history of each other. In other words, when the nurse enters into the other's experience a new energetic phenomenal *Caritas Field* is created that is greater than the two persons; thus another person enters into the nurse's experience. This shared experience creates its own energetic phenomenal field and becomes part of a larger, deeper, complex pattern of life.

ART OF TRANSPERSONAL CARING

According to Tolstoy (1975), if one ponders the meaning of art, one must first consider that art is a condition of human life and a means of human-to-human contact. The human-to-human contact causes the receiver of art to enter into a certain kind of relationship, both with the creator of art and with all those who simultaneously, previously, or subsequently receive the same or similar artistic expression. Another special feature of art is that feelings are transmitted.

The activity of art is based on the fact that a person receiving another person's expression of feeling, through hearing, sight, or even intuition, is capable of experiencing the emotion that moved the other to express it. One person's level of humanity and experience is reflected onto another. To use the simplest example, one person laughs and another who hears it becomes merry, or a person weeps and another who hears it feels sorrow. If a man is excited or irritated, another who sees him may develop a similar state of mind. By his movements or by the sounds of his voice, a person expresses courage and determination, anger or calmness, and this state of mind passes on to others. A person suffers, manifesting his suffering by groans and spasms, and this suffering transmits itself to other people; a woman expresses her feelings of admiration, devotion, fear, respect, or love of certain persons, objects, or phenomena, and others are moved by the same feelings of admiration, devotion, fear, respect, or love, to the same persons, objects, or phenomena.

It is on this capacity of one human being to receive another human being's expression of feeling and to experience those feelings for one's self that the artistic activity of nursing and caring is based. The art of caring in nursing begins when the nurse, with the object of joining another (or others) to one's self with a certain feeling of caring, compassion, and concern, expresses that feeling by certain inner and external indications.

Art is not just moving another directly and immediately by giving vent to feelings at the very time they are experienced. If a person causes another to relax, cry, or laugh when he himself is obliged to laugh or cry, that does not amount to the art of caring. It is art when the nurse, having experienced or realized the feelings of another, is able to detect and sense these feelings and in turn is able to express them in such a way that the other person is able to experience them more fully and release the feelings he or she has been longing to express.

The feelings that the nurse as an artist inculcates in others may be varied—strong or weak, important or insignificant. They may be feelings of love, fear, courage, joy, quietness, awe. It is all art.

The activity of the art and artistry of caring in nursing is triggered by the human interaction in a nursing care situation. The human-to-human process evokes within the nurse a feeling. Having experienced that feeling and having evoked it in one's self, then by means of movements, touch, sounds, words, colors, and forms, the nurse transmits the feeling so that another person experiences the same feeling—that is the activity of the art and artistry of transpersonal human caring.

The art of transpersonal caring is a human activity consisting of the following: A nurse consciously, by means of certain signs, nonverbal expressions, consciousness, intentionality, and heart-centered loving healing presence, passes on to others feelings he or she has lived through, realized, or learned. Others are united by these feelings and also experience them. The chief peculiarity of this feeling is that the recipient of a truly artistic caring impression is so united to the nurse's expression that he or she feels the feeling as his or her own, to the degree that what is expressed is just what he or she had been longing and wishing to express. A truly caring nurse/artist is able to eliminate in the consciousness of the recipient the separation between him- or herself and the nurse. In other words, the nurse is able to form a union, a deeply human-to-human spirit-to-spirit connection with the other person on a level that transcends the physical and that preserves the subjectivity and physicality of persons without reducing them to the moral status of objects. As such, there is a freeing of both persons from their separation and isolation, in this uniting, of the feeling with another and with others who have also experienced the same feelings. The union of feelings can potentiate self-healing, discovery of inner power, and control and contribute to another finding meaning in his or her existence. That is the great attractive force of the art and human artistry of transpersonal caring–healing in nursing and all healthcare practices.

If the nurse is able to detect accurately the other's condition of soul, if he or she feels this emotion, and this union with another, and in turn can express it accurately, then the recipient has a release of the feeling he or she has been longing and wishing to express; thus, human subjectivity is restored. This is what I call the art of transpersonal caring. If, however, there has been no such awareness, no union of the feelings of the moment that are moved by the human caring process, then transpersonal caring has not occurred. I view this act of transpersonal caring in nursing as a human art, a human caring science, and a moral ideal of nursing.

Premises

The more individual and authentic the feelings are that the nurse conveys, the more strongly does the caring process affect the recipient. The more individual the state of soul is that is transferred, the more release, satisfaction, pleasure, and peace does the recipient obtain, and the more readily and strongly does another experience the caring and join in it. In other words, the full use of the self is called on in this level of caring–healing (*Caritas*) nursing (Watson, 2008).

A clarity of expression assists the nurse's caring. The more clearly the feeling is communicated (which the other has long known and felt at some level but which is now realized more fully, and for which expression has only now been found), the better able is the recipient to experience the union.

Most of all, the degree of transpersonal caring (in this sense of unity of feeling and spirit-to-spirit connection) is increased by the degree of authenticity and individual sincerity of the nurse. If the recipient believes the nurse is contriving the feelings and has not actually felt a union with the condition of the other's soul but is "going through the process," trying to act on the other's feelings, and does not feel within his- or herself what longs to be expressed, resistance immediately springs up. Trust is violated and superficial responses result. Thereafter, the most unique response, elaborate approach, and the cleverest techniques not only fail to release but actually repel another person and contribute to the state of disharmony (illness).

The authenticity and the individuality go together, because if the nurse is authentic he or she will be able to express the feeling as he or she experiences or realizes it in his or her own authentic way in a given moment. It cannot be sugar-coated over as a distant, professional clinical script often introduced these days to address patient satisfaction and institutional scores. Because every nurse is a unique person, his or her feelings will be individual. The more individual they are, the more the nurse as artist has drawn them from the depths of his or her nature, and the more natural and authentic they will be. The condition of authenticity and sincerity has always been complied with in peasant art and nature, and this helps explain why such acts and arts are so powerful.

However, it is a condition that is almost entirely absent in our educational and socializing experiences in the nursing profession and is instead substituted with artificial aims of clinical–medical views of humanity through professionalism and scientism. Such are the conditions of transpersonal caring that help to decide the artistic expression of the human caring process in nursing, which as a moral ideal is considered apart from the facts of the subject. Indeed, the art and artistry of transpersonal caring help to mediate between facts and meaning, helping others to find right-relation, more harmony, more healing, more options for self-control, self-knowledge, self-caring, and self-healing.

Each one of the above-mentioned conditions may vary. For one nurse, for example, the level of spirituality, creativity, and individuality of the feeling transmitted may predominate; for another nurse, clarity of expression; for a third, sincerity and authenticity; whereas a fourth may have sincerity and individuality but may be deficient in clarity; a fifth may have individuality and clarity but less sincerity; and so forth, to all possible degrees and in all combinations. The union between the nurse and recipient of care allows for both to have an intimate relationship with their spiritual selves.

Likewise, the nurse, through spirituality, creativity, individuality, clarity, and authentic self, may draw on various combinations of expression of feelings. One may rely more on acts and movements; another on words, senses, and sounds; another on presence, silence and nonverbal expression; and still another on precision, forms, or information, knowledge, or color, intentional touch, and so forth, again to all possible degrees and in all possible combinations. Thus, it is true for the nurse and thus true for the recipient regarding the possible degrees and combinations with which one communicates the condition of the soul. As Mary Catherine Bateson (Margaret Mead's daughter) related, every act is practiced improvisation in that no two moments can ever be the same. Each human-to-human connection is a once in a lifetime encounter and can never be repeated. Yet, what happens in that moment informs the next moment and so on; we carry these moments for the rest of our life, for better or for worse, affecting our depth of feeling and options to deepen our very humanity and meaningful human existence.

SUMMARY OF TRANSPERSONAL CARING

The art and artistry of transpersonal caring as a moral ideal are a means of communication and release of human feelings through the coparticipation of one's entire self in nursing. Transpersonal caring therefore is a means of progress in which an individual moves toward a higher/deeper sense of self and harmony, evolving in consciousness to a higher level of self in relation to that which is greater than self.

Collectively, the art of transpersonal caring allows humanity to move toward greater harmony, spiritual evolution, and omega point/perfection. Such a union of feelings and caring communication renders accessible to humans all the knowledge and experience discovered through the expression of, and reflection upon, preceding generations and ancestors, as well as people in one's own time. The art of transpersonal caring in nursing makes accessible to a person a sense of common humanity across time and space. It awakens intersubjectivity experienced historically, globally, and culturally by our ancestors, mythologies, belief systems, values of other peoples, and civilizations, as well as our contemporaries in similar human conditions.

As the evolution of human thought progresses with the addition of truer and more necessary knowledge/wisdom, dislodging and replacing what was mistaken and unnecessary, so the evolution of human feelings and human consciousness shift can proceed toward a moral community of caring, by means of the moral ideal of transpersonal caring in all human-to-human relations; whereby feelings less kind and less necessary for the well-being of humankind can be replaced by kinder, loving, connecting, and more necessary feelings for the well-being and dignity and even the survival of humankind and Mother Earth planet. This shift makes explicit that there is a relation between human caring and peace in our world. This human honoring process is the value of the art of transpersonal caring in nursing, moving in concentric circles, from self, to other, to community, to Planet Earth all the way out into the infinity of the universe. The more the art of transpersonal caring in nursing advances the kinder, more loving, and more helpful feelings for the human, the more evolved is one's caring consciousness, and we can define ideal caring with reference to its content and subject matter of nursing.

In the idea of transpersonal nursing, as developed through the study of Tolstoy's work, there is room for art, science, ethics, technology, and metaphysics. With our attention to the vicissitudes of humanity, caring artistry along with intersubjective feelings, and the authentic individuality of each situation, the process allows for combinations of expressions of human feelings in different moments and contexts and with different outcomes that can never be fully explained or predicted.

The emphasis on the deeply human component of feelings and human-to-human caring is consistent with my view of the person. Transpersonal caring not only allows for release of emotions and the evolution of the person's spiritual self or soul, but it promotes congruence between the person's perception and experience and promotes self as is and one's higher self, potentiating harmony and healing. The process allows the nurse to reflect the self back on the self.

The transpersonal caring process is largely art and human artistry because of the way it touches another person's soul and feels the emotion and union with another, the goal being the movement of the person toward a higher sense of self and a greater sense of harmony. In turn, the process contributes to the movement of humans toward perfection/de Chardin's view of omega point, which contributes to the sustainability and preservation of humanity.

The union of the two persons in which the condition of the human soul and feelings have been transmitted allows for liberation of the human mind, spirit, and soul that leads to a greater sense of strength, power, and human capacity for finding the purposive and metaphorical meanings in existence and illness. It also establishes an intimate relationship with one's spiritual self through the artistic human caring connections.

The transpersonal caring of the nurse in which the feelings are released allows the one being cared for to assimilate better the condition of one's soul into his or her self. The assimilation may lead to some reorganization or re-patterning of one's self as perceived and one's self as experienced. Both will be more unified, which is in essence what each one is spiritually already.

The context for viewing the person and the nurse in the theory of transpersonal caring is in the moment-to-moment human spirit-to-spirit connection between the two people. The coming together of the two—one the caregiver and the other the care receiver—comprises an event. An event connotes an actual caring occasion in which intersubjective caring moments can occur.

The person's consciousness, intentionality, authentic presence, and emotions then become the starting point, the focal point, and the point of access to the soul and the body. Once the person moves toward a higher sense of self with increased harmony, then one's own self-healing processes and one's capacity for finding meaning in existence are available. At that point one can better choose between health/healing and illness, regardless of any disease or bodily or human condition.

It is not so much the what of the nursing acts or even the caring connections per se, it is the how (the relation between the what and the how), the transpersonal nature and presence of the union of two persons' soul(s), that allows for some unknowns to emerge from the caring itself.

The ideas expressed here about transpersonal caring–healing as a moral ideal for nursing allow nurses to call on the inner depth of their own humanness and personal creativity as they realize the conditions of a person's soul and their own. The intersubjective process of caring–healing is infinite and will continue to expand as knowledge and approaches expand. The transpersonal human-to-human caring is the essence and moral ideal of a style of nursing where human dignity and humanity are preserved and human indignity is alleviated in health–illness experiences.

REFERENCES

Gadow, S. (1980). Existential advocacy: Philosophical foundation of nursing. In S. Spieker & S. Gadow (Eds.), *Nursing images and ideals* (pp. 86–101). New York: Springer.

Tart, C. (Ed.). (1976). *Transpersonal psychologies*. New York: Harper & Row.

Tolstoy, L. (1975). What is art? (L. & A. Maude, trans.) In J. Hersey (Ed.), *The writer's craft* (pp. 25–30). New York: Knopf.

CHAPTER 9

Structural Overview of Watson's Theory of Human Care

SYNOPSIS

Subject Matter

The primary subject matter of this theory is as follows:

1. Human caring as humanitarian science and art, which requires ongoing explication and development, cannot be assumed.
2. Human caring science provides the philosophical-ethical-epistemic-ontological disciplinary foundation to sustain nursing and its covenant with society/humankind.
3. A unitary transformative world view orientation toward humanity and role in the universe.
4a. Mutuality of both nurse and patient as one gestalt and transpersonal energetic *Caritas* phenomenal field in a given moment; the nurse–patient relationship occurs within a context of intersubjectivity.
4b. A unitary world view of connectedness of all.
5. Human caring relationship in nursing as a moral ideal, a consciousness, an intentionality that includes concepts such as energetic *Caritas*

Core Aspects: Caring Science Theory of Human Caring

- Relational Caring as Ethical-Moral-Philosophical Values-Guided Foundation
- Caring Core: 10 Carative Factors/Caritas Processes—Love-Heart-Centered Caring/Compassion
- Transpersonal Caring Moment—The Caritas Field
- Caring as Consciousness—Energy-Intertionality—Heart-Centered Human Presence
- Caring–Healing Modalities

phenomenal field, actual caring occasion, caring moment, and transpersonal caring–healing.

6. Human caring as both immanent and transcendent in a given moment and inviting a return to metaphysics in our life and science world.

Also inherent within the subject matter are the notions of health–illness, environment, and universe and how they interact, intersect, and transcend the physical–material objects and values of life. This human caring science disciplinary foundation invites the return of love and the heart-centered human as the evolved practitioner of caring–healing (*Caritas* Nursing* Watson, 2008).

Values

The values inherent in this work are associated with deep respect and openness for the wonders, mysteries, and even miracles of life and the power of humans to change and evolve to a higher/deeper level of consciousness. In the views of Teilhard de Chardin, one wants to evolve toward the omega point, to become more godly, more holy, more divine, more in line with one's spiritual destiny, dignity, and one's *soul's code.*

There is an underlying value for the highest regard and reverence for the spiritual–inner subjective life world—the spirit-filled person with power to grow and change; a human-to-human mutually relating, authentic caring–healing presence approach to helping a person gain more self-knowledge, self-caring, self-control, and self-healing, regardless of the presenting health–illness life-challenging situation or condition. For example, one may be cured, but not healed; on the other hand, someone may not be cured but experience an ultimate healing through peaceful dying/death, returning to spirit/mystery. This underlying value system of this theory is blended with the language and structure of the original theoretical constructs: the 10 carative factors (Watson, 1979, 1985), such as humanistic–altruism values, sensitivity to self and others, and a love for a trust of life and other humans. More recently these expanded to include the evolved theory of 10 caritas processes, acknowledging the practice of heart-centered loving kindness, compassion, and equanimity; creative solution-seeking (versus focusing on problems per se) through

---

*Interventions is used in categorizing nursing theory and components of a nursing model in the literature. The term "intervention" sounds harsh and mechanical and is inconsistent with my ideas and ideals. A more consistent term for my purposes might be caring–healing modalities and nursing therapeutics. I have reframed interventions as such.

From Watson's work, *Nursing: The Philosophy and Science of Caring* (Boston: Little, Brown, 1979). Slight changes are made in the language of the carative factors, especially to number 6.

embracing all ways of knowing for human caring practices and caring modalities; and even allowing for miracles and existential/spiritual mysteries to unfold. Finally, human caring is honored as a moral ideal of nursing with a conscious intentionality and compassionate concern for preservation of humanity, dignity, preservation of integrity, and wholeness of self/other on one's inner and outer life journey.

Goals

The goals for the theory ideals are associated with the evolving heart-centered human, honoring mental–spiritual growth and evolving consciousness to higher, deeper awareness for self and others, finding meaning in one's own suffering, existence and experiences, discovering inner power and control, and potentiating instances of transcendence and self-healing.

Caring–Healing Modalities: Nursing Therapeutics

The interventions in this theory are reframed as caring–healing modalities and nursing therapeutics. They are related to the human caring–healing process with full participation of the nurse/person with the patient/person.** Human caring requires knowledge of human caring–healing consciousness, presence and processes, and caring competencies/literacy to balance and complement the medical/technological competencies and skills. Caring requires knowledge and understanding of individual needs; knowledge of how to respond to others' needs; knowledge of our strengths and limitations; knowledge of who the other person is, his or her strengths and limitations, and the meaning of the situation for him or her; and knowledge of how to comfort, and offer compassion and authentic presence; and to hold another in his or her wholeness, while he or she is vulnerable, hurt, wounded and suffering. Human caring also requires enabling actions, that is, actions that allow another to seek creative solutions to life situations, to grow, evolve, and transcend the here and now, actions that are related to general and specific knowledge and practices of caring and healing.

The caring–healing modalities related to the human caring process require a consciousness, an intentionality, a will, a mutual relating, and actions. This process entails a commitment to human caring as a moral ideal directed toward the preservation of humanity and sustaining human caring in instances where it is threatened, biologically or otherwise. The process affirms the subjectivity of persons and the intersubjective connection between the nurse and patient and helps to facilitate right-relation for self/other while allowing evolving consciousness and spiritual growth. The structure and language of the caring theory and naming of the phenomenon of human caring are found in the original carative factors (Watson, 1979, 1985) and the new transposed language from 10 carative factors to 10 caritas processes (**Watson, 2008).

All these carative factors/caritas processes become actualized in the moment-to-moment human caring process in which the nurse is being with the other person (whether administering an emergency intravenous treatment to a critical care patient or changing the linen of an unconscious patient). Human caring requires the nurse to possess a caring consciousness, an intentionality, and a healing presence along with the will, values, and commitment to an ideal of intersubjective human-to-human caring moments that are directed toward the preservation of personhood, dignity, and humanity of both nurse and patient. Although these are ideals, different nurses and different moments allow higher levels of caring. The degree of caring is influenced by multiple, complex dynamics and patterns. The more human caring is actualized as a mutual experience and intersubjective connection in each caring moment, the more potential the caring holds for human health-healing goals to be met through finding meaning in one's own existence, discovering one's own inner power and control, and potentiating instances of transcendence and self-healing.

Common Human Tasks

These human caring experiences parallel common tasks we share as humans on this Earth plane journey (Watson, 2008):

- Learning to heal our relationship with self and other, and Mother Nature/Earth
- Transforming human suffering and/or finding meaning in suffering
- Deepening our understanding of meaning of life and acceptance of all its ups and downs with compassion and equanimity
- Deepening our understanding and acceptance of impermanence, of death/dying as part of the sacred circle of life
- Preparing for our own death
- Remembering why we are here on the Earth plane
- Questioning: What are our gifts and talents? Why are we here? What are we here to fulfill as our Earth purpose? What is our soul's journey and destiny on this sacred life journey?

**Transposed Caritas processes: From Watson's 2008 book, *Nursing: The Philosophy and Science of Caring. New revised edition.* (Boulder, CO: University Press of Colorado).

Finally, the human caring science/human caring theory allows nursing individually and collectively to contribute to the preservation of humanity in an individual, in society, and in civilization globally. These moral ideals for human-to-human caring foster the spiritual evolution of humankind toward a global moral community of caring and peace.

Perspective

The perspective is spiritual–existential and phenomenological in orientation, but it also draws on some indigenous practices, Eastern philosophy, evolved Western beliefs, and ancient wisdom traditions across time. Many of the principles and premises are consistent with the blueprint of Nightingale, which have yet to be actualized in this 21st century.

Context

The context is humanitarian, ethically scientific, and metaphysical. It incorporates both the art and science of nursing. Science is emphasized in an expanded model of science that incorporates the human, caring, and love. Thus, it introduces an evolving view of a humanitarian science as the disciplinary foundation of nursing.

Approach

The approach is globally descriptive within an evolving worldview shift; the moral–ethical, ontological–cosmological ideals have been described as possibly prescriptive, clarifying the value-laden human-covenantal, disciplinary foundation of nursing as human caring science.

Method

The optimal method for studying the theory is more naturally through field study that is qualitative in design. My views are most congruent with phenomenological–existential interpretive, creative forms of inquiry and evolving methodologies for study and research. The ideas also allow for an applied humanities or applied philosophy or ethics approach. A word of caution regarding method is that there is no consensus regarding one scientific method.

It depends on what components of the theory or what phenomenon one chooses to research. The best rule of thumb is that the method should fit the phenomena under study; one should not force a phenomenon of interest into a scientific method when there is an acknowledged need for alternative or new methods, and vice versa.

I am supportive of a range of conventional and exploratory methods and encourage scholars to pursue a creative-paradigm-transcending approach that fits with a new philosophy of science while maintaining high standards, rigor, and credibility. Examples are historical research, comparative case/care studies, narrative and story, textual hermeneutic analysis, photographic–artistic documentaries, literary works, philosophical analysis, and subjecting clinical data to new analytic techniques, such as empirical phenomenological analysis, poetics, dramatic performance pieces, movement/dance, neo-ethnographic approaches, and so on.

REFERENCES

Watson, J. (1979, 1985). *Nursing: The philosophy and science of caring.* Boston: Little, Brown. Reprinted 1985, Boulder, CO: University Press of Colorado.

Watson, J. (2008). *Nursing: The philosophy and science of caring. New revised edition.* Boulder, CO: University Press of Colorado.

BIBLIOGRAPHY

American Nurses Association. (1980). *Social policy statement.* Kansas City, MO: Author.

Gadow, S. (1984). Existential advocacy as a form of caring: Technology, truth and touch. Paper presented to Research Seminar Series: The Development of Nursing as a Human Science. School of Nursing, University of Colorado Health Sciences Center, Denver, March.

Watson, J. (1979). *Nursing: The philosophy and science of caring.* Boston: Little, Brown. Reprinted 1985. Boulder, CO: University Press of Colorado.

CHAPTER 10

Methodology: Reconsidered

*"Once we seek ontological and epistemological authenticity with the
methodologies for studying human experiences, then we must
consider authentic language to capture the experience . . .
—the result may be poetizing."*

—JEAN WATSON (1994, P. 14)

The methodologies for studying transpersonal caring and developing nursing as a human caring science and art require an expanded view of science and reside in methods that are based on different assumptions about the

- Nature of reality: unitary, context, relational dependent
- Nature of inquirer–object–subject relationship: relationship and inquiry process is part of the field on influence
- Nature of truth statements: multiple truths, findings are context dependent, generating new hypotheses for understanding depth of a human phenomenon
- Nature of phenomenon under study: method should fit the nature of phenomenon
- View of science: product or process discovery; paradigm adherence or paradigm transcending

ONTOLOGICAL AND EPISTEMOLOGICAL AUTHENTICITY

Other aspects of methods that need to be considered for relevance to study of human experiences and caring–healing processes have to do with aspects of trustworthiness of the data (for example, truth value or confidence in findings), applicability, consistency, and neutrality. Moreover, one has to consider various other dimensions related to method such as quality criterion, theory source, knowledge types, instruments, design, and setting. Authenticity of language is another consideration with respect to human caring methods; it is significant to use language that captures the embedded human meanings and expressions— allowing for evocative, metaphoric, even poetic language to accurately express and convey/communicate human life experiences (Watson, 1987; Chinn and Watson, 1994).

The methodologies that are relevant for studying my theory can be classified generally as qualitative–naturalistic–phenomenological field and interpretive, expressive methods of inquiry or a combined qualitative–quantitative inquiry versus a quantitative rationalistic method of inquiry as the exclusive method.

The nursing theory of transpersonal caring (within the framework of qualitative–phenomenological–naturalistic approach) can use a variety of qualitative/quantitative, creative methods for exploring meanings of human existence, illness, human caring, and human capacities for healing. These include earlier descriptive approaches such as existential case studies and content analysis; other methods for consideration include ethno methodology (a phenomenological approach used at the social–cultural level).

EXPANDED EPISTEMOLOGICAL METHODS

Once we concur that nursing and human phenomenon incorporate multiple ways of knowing and being, then it invites and evokes multiple ways to reveal human experiential phenomenon in authentic ways and approaches. One of the more popular and prominent methods that has evolved over the past couple of decades and is increasingly being acknowledged as an appropriate method for nursing by a number of nursing theorists and researchers is the henomenological/hermeneutic/interpretive forms of inquiry, including narrative and story as method. Because most of the other qualitative approaches in some way or other are phenomenological, it is worthy of further development.

As an interlude one is referred to the Appendix, which includes an early exemplar of two phenomenological approaches used in making sense of the findings when studying loss and grief among an Aboriginal community in a Western Australia outback reserve. It serves only as an example. However, it is important to point out that these and other methods are in need of further development and practice, whereas new creative methods are constantly being explored around the world. Nurses are encouraged to create new approaches that are appropriate for the phenomena under study. For now I confine my work to expanded notions of the phenomenological method and my views on its relevance and evolution as method for human caring science and transpersonal caring. It is only one approach.

Expanded Phenomenological Methodology

This conventional view of phenomenological method consists of describing or explicating experience in the language of experience that captures the authenticity of the human feelings. The method attempts to describe and understand human experiences as they appear in awareness and from within the subjective world of the person/and the intersubjective emergence of findings from the experience. These experiences can include phenomenon such as human caring–healing, but also experiences related to human health and illness conditions, such as loss–grieving, anxiety, hope, despair, love, suffering, loneliness, spiritual self, higher sense of consciousness, and an almost infinity of human experiences and concepts of existence. In brief, the subject matter of phenomenological research is human experiences—their types and their structures, along with their inner subjective meaning, expressions, essence, and relationships.

Husserl, considered the father of phenomenology, was concerned that a phenomenological analysis of experiences should not be confused with a psychological analysis of experiences (1977). Psychology is viewed in this sense as an empirical science that studies experiences as empirical events in an empirical world, with all its descriptions and generalizations referring to experiences in this empirical context.

Husserl's (1977) idea of phenomenology involved a different attitude: It involved *placing within brackets* the existential, *historical* aspect of experiences and concentrating on the *essence* or the *ideal types* exemplified by the experiences that we either have or are able to conceive of ourselves as having. Phenomenology studies such essences and clarifies the various relationships between them. Heidegger's (1962) point of view was that experiences that merit the greatest philosophical attention are those that find expression in poetry. He believed that only through a searching phenomenological analysis of experiences could we hope to achieve a clarification of the meaning of being.

Human phenomena (such as caring, caring moments, and events of being, that is, illness, health) are not object-like; they cannot be inspected or studied in the manner of objects. They have to do with the "how" rather than the "what." They are not neutral items that call for a neutral and detached independent description. They have to do with modes of existing and the meaning of being. The human phenomena of nursing make themselves known through moods, feelings, and emotions of experiences.

Although there are different views regarding the course that phenomenological research should pursue and the principal objectives of such research, what unites the different views is an acceptance of the general principle that priority should be given to an analysis of experiences from the point of view of those who have the experiences or are able to have them. Even though there are gradually more and more objections about the traditional, rationalistic, quantitative methodologies for human caring science, and specifically nursing science, it is still difficult to transform those objections into a concrete research program.

Some of the early work of Professor Amedeo Giorgi of Duquesne University, Pittsburgh (Giorgi, 1975), and the research group at the Department of Education at the University of Goteborg, Sweden, historically elaborated on an empirical approach that is phenomenological. From their point of view the contribution of phenomenology as a method was that it offered an alternative way of looking at the investigation of human phenomena.

Merleau-Ponty's ideas (1964) also have important considerations for nursing. According to Merleau-Ponty, the key to understanding phenomenology was to take, as a given, that humans behave but to give human behavior its "proper ontological status," that is, to take it out of the purely physical domain. Merleau-Ponty then conceptualized behavior as a relation between the subject and the world, where the relationship is a dialectic one. Consequently, any human phenomena are in a subject–world relation because embodied in the concept is the idea that the person is necessarily conscious of "something" and thereby directed toward the world. The acknowledgment of the unity of subject–world relationship allows the possibility of our being able to be faithful to the experience of the world as subjectively viewed. We can describe neither the objective nor the subjective world but only the world as we experience it.

To allow for the inseparability of subject–world, it is important to make a distinction between different levels of attending to (being in) the world (Alexandersson, 1981). At one level we are handling the world in a prereflective manner, which means we are close to it, directly involved in it, and living it. In Merleau-Ponty's words, "I am outside myself in the world of my project" (1964, pp. 186 and 187).

However, an experience embodies a dialogue between subject and world and suggests something more than just the world we direct our attention to at the prereflective level. If we are to be able to attend to something else, for example, the way of experiencing, to attending to that which is beyond self in the larger universe, then we need a second level of attending, called the reflective level. Thus, at the reflective level the object of an investigation is the relation between what is experienced (for example, human caring) and how it is experienced (Merleau-Ponty, 1964). At some level of understanding, phenomenology emerged as a method to explore existential (spiritual) phenomena, which are difficult to capture in conventional methods.

According to European perspectives from Giorgi (1970), Alexandersson (1981), Marton (1981), and Zaner (1975), experienced at conducting ground breaking, early pioneering phenomenological research, the key to phenomenology as a method is that we take into account the way the world is experienced; this requires phenomenological *reduction*. It consists of considering not only what is experienced, existentially and even spiritually, but the mode or manner in which it is experienced.

In Alexandersson's (1981) view, this reduction is not reductionistic in conventional science notions; rather it is to take a step back from our experience, reflect upon it, then explore reflectively on what is the structure underneath the experience; what was the structure of the experience which allowed it to occur? According to Zaner (1975), phenomenology's chief method is that of reduction. He explains phenomenological reduction in terms of "shifts of focal attention" and consequent "reflective orientations."

It is important to highlight again, that phenomenological reduction is not at all akin to what has come to be known as reductivism (for example, in philosophy of science); it has nothing whatsoever to do with any attempt to simplify or economize, much less to try to explain one region by showing it to be reducible to another. Rather, "the basic thrust is found in the literal meaning of the term 'reduction': a leading back to origins, beginnings, which have become obscure, hidden, or covered over by other things" (Zaner, 1975, p. 126).

The phenomenological reduction in no way denies what is naturally believed in or posited by our natural consciousness but rather is a deliberate effort to "suspend" or "put in abeyance" that attitude to examine it in depth. The reduction, then, is the systematic effort to bring the natural attitude into focus by considering not only what is experienced but how it is experienced.

The phenomenological reduction method is a six-step procedure:

1. The experience is bracketed/suspended/regarded as an appearance (one seeks to hold one's own perception and judgments in abeyance, as much as possible, while simultaneously being mindful of one's own inner processes; this process includes mindfulness to catch one's self in the process, being able to empty out assumptions in order to be authentically present, "hear" the deep meaning from other's expression and reported experience).

2. The experienced phenomenon is imaginatively varied to obtain the invariant feature of the phenomenon—to discuss the necessary structure of the experience or the essence of phenomenon.

3. The experience is mirrored back onto the researcher as he or she immerses him- or herself to find the deep meaning in the experience/phenomenon.

4. The researcher thus becomes part of the interpretation and thus forms of creative scholarship, i.e., imaginative, artistic, inspired, metaphorical, poetic insight emerges, which often transcends the original data, thus offering new understanding and meaning to capture the essence of the phenomenon.

5. This subject-to-subject engagement of the researcher with the data and phenomenon can generate discovery of new insights/essence of "knowing" (intersubjective confirmability) through the form of expressive/interpretive

inquiry. The researcher is seeking ontological and epistemological authenticity with the human experience/phenomenon in question.

6. The result in turn seeks to find authentic language to capture the experience. It may be metaphorical, poetic, and artistic in expression.

TRANSCENDENTAL PHENOMENOLOGY: POETICIZING AS TRUTH*

What is truth in research? In Gadamer's (1991) *Truth and Method,* he sought to show the drawbacks of methodology's rule with the human sciences. He turned to the arts and poetry to gain access to a truth more irresistible than that offered by sometimes dogmatic applications of methods.

Parker Palmer (1987) reminded us to be careful with our development of knowledge and truth because we shape souls with the shape of our knowledge. Perhaps in a human caring science context for method, we understand that truth is not necessarily discovered *without* but by engagement and interpretation and deep meaning seeking.

I was stuck recently when I heard a policy panel discussion on television when one of the speakers reminded the panel, "There are facts, and then there is the truth." So we do not necessarily obtain the truth via facts alone. Nurses have a dominant role in mediating constantly between medical-scientific-technical facts and meaning they hold for the experiences of the patient, family, and loved ones. As Polanyi (1962) suggested, facts have to go through an authentication process before they can be shown to be 'scientific.' Because we are humans caring for others in life crises and change, our truths are cocreated through a process of values and meaning, making through language. There is no one Truth with a capital T, but multiple truths, depending upon the experiencing and perceiving human.

As Gadamer (1991) explained, the current ontological shift toward hermeneutics is guided by language; words hold meaning and authentic interpretations. We have no choice of not seeing truth, of not knowing, because it is the nature of being human to formulate meanings to have some sense of truth within our world and within ourselves.

The concept of capturing the authentic experience and essence does not necessarily mean literal expression. It does not mean absolute, definite, and beyond cultural dependencies but more pragmatically represents the deepest understanding available, established on the basis of intersubjective agreement

---

*This section draws upon Watson (1994, pp. 3–17).

and ontological-epistemological consistency and congruence of a given context. Intersubjectivity consists of having others independently describe a phenomenon as experienced and reported and then comparing the results. Intersubjectivity also means there is subjective congruence, authenticity of capturing the phenomenon; finding alignment with the findings that are internally, experientially, and subjectively validated by others. Thus, there is "intersubjective confirmability" between and among the findings, in contrast with objective validation from outer. Often, this result is poeticizing; indeed, it cannot be other than poetic. As Levin (1981, in Watson, 1994, p. 14) expressed it:

> In phenomenological discourse, the deepest transcendental truth of an existentially authentic languaging of experience will be articulated naturally with the sensuous resonance, the emotional spaciousness and the elemental openness of the poetic word. Heidegger has recommended that we create an authenticity whereby the experiences speak for themselves. IN the process the researcher is transformed by their participation, true to a moving human experience which evokes mutuality of both parties.

In other words, how could cold, unfeeling, detached, dogmatic words and tone possibly reveal the truth or depth of meaning of a human phenomenon associated with transpersonal caring–healing associated with sorrow, suffering, loss, change, along with great beauty, passion, compassion, joy, and so on (Watson, 1994)? Words and language that are bereft of feelings of loving kindness, gentleness, caring, compassion, or forgiveness lack congruence and authenticity.

In summary, the phenomenological method in all its configurations and evolutions seeks to invite the human and authentic human experiences, and languaging of human phenomenon, back into the research methods. This perspective represents a most contemporary postmodern turn in human caring science method. It shifts the focus from facts and numbers alone to meaning, story, connections, understanding, and authentic expressions through a variety of creative scholarship: metaphor, poetry, art, music, drama, performance or other forms that continue to evolve. Thus, new knowledge/understanding and language are revealed about a deeply human expressive phenomenon in which the researcher is a coparticipant. Finally, as this one explored method, within human caring science context, continues to deepen and evolve, we reconnect with who and what we have become/are becoming as humans: cocreators of ourselves and our discipline of nursing as art and science. Hopefully we discover an old/new place in which we can dwell as humanitarian and scientific scholars.

REFERENCES

Alexandersson, C. (1981). Amedeo Giorgi's empirical phenomenology (publication no. 3). Swedish Council for Research in Humanities and Social Sciences, Department of Education, University of Goteborg, Sweden.

Chinn, P. L., & Watson, J. (Eds.). (1994). *Art and aesthetics in nursing.* New York: National League for Nursing.

Gadamer, H. G. (1991). Truth and method (2nd rev. ed.). New York: Crossroad Publishing.

Giorgi, A. (1970). *Psychology as a human science: A phenomenologically based approach.* New York: Harper & Row.

Giorgi, A. (1975). An application of phenomenological method in psychology. In A. Giorgi, C. Fisher, & E. Murray (Eds.), *Duquesne studies in phenomenological psychology* (vol. 2, pp. 82–104). Pittsburgh, PA: Duquesne University Press.

Heidegger, M. (1962). *Being and time.* New York: Harper & Row.

Husserl, E. (1977). *Phenomenological psychology* (pp. 20–45). The Hague, Netherlands: Martinus Nijhoff.

Levin, D. (1983). The poetic function in phenomenological discourse. In W. McBride & C. Schrag (Eds.), *Phenomenology in a pluralistic context.* Albany, NY: State University of New York Press.

Merleau-Ponty, M. (1964). *The primacy of perception.* Evanston, IL: Northwestern University Press.

Palmer, P. (1987). Community, conflict and ways of knowing. *Magazine of Higher Education, 19,* 20–25.

Polanyi, M. (1962). *Personal knowledge.* New York: Harper & Row.

Watson, J. (1987). Nursing on the caring edge. Metaphorical vignettes. *Advances in Nursing Science, 10*(1), 10–18.

Watson, J. (1994). Poeticizing as truth through language. In P. Chinn & J. Watson (Eds.), *Art and aesthetics in nursing* (pp. 3–17). New York: National League for Nursing.

Zaner, R. (1975). On the sense of method of phenomenology. In E. Pivcevic (Ed.), *Phenomenology and philosophical understanding* (125–140). London: Cambridge University Press.

BIBLIOGRAPHY

Alexandersson, C. (1981). Amedeo Giorgi's empirical phenomenology. (publication no. 3). Swedish Council for Research in Humanities and Social Sciences, Department of Education, University of Goteborg, Sweden.

Barret, W. (1962). *Irrational man.* New York: Doubleday.

Betteridge, H. T. (Ed.). (1958). *The new Cassell's German dictionary.* New York: Funk and Wagnals.

Binswanger, L. (1958). Insanity as life-historical phenomenon and as mental disease: The case of Ilse. In R. May, E. Angel, & H. I. Ellenberger (Eds.), *Existence.* New York: Basic Books.

Boss, M. (1963). *Psychoanalysis and daseinsanalysis.* New York: Basic Books.

Buber, M. (1958). *I and Thou* (2nd ed.). New York: Scribners.

Capra, F. (1982). *The turning point.* New York: Simon & Schuster.

Davis, A. J. (1978). The phenomenological approach in nursing research. In N. Chaska (Ed.), *The nursing profession: Views through the mist.* New York: McGraw-Hill.

Dennis, N. (1982). Personal communication and health seminar, Western Australian Institute of Technology, Australia.

Frankl, V. E. (1963). *Man's search for meaning.* New York: Washington Square Press.

Frye, N. (1964). *The educated imagination.* Bloomington, IN: Indiana University Press.

Giorgi, A. (1975). An application of phenomenological method in psychology. In A. Giorgi, C. Fisher, & E. Murray (Eds.), *Duquesne Studies in Phenomenological Psychology* (vol. 2). Pittsburgh, PA: Duquesne University Press.

Giorgi, A. (1970). *Psychology as a human science: A phenomenologically based approach.* New York: Harper & Row.

Hall, C. S., & Lindzey, F. (1978). *Theories of Personality* (3rd ed.). New York: Wiley.

Heelan, P. (1977). Hermeneutics of experimental science in the context of life-world. In D. Ihde & R. Zaner (Eds.), *Interdisciplinary Phenomenology.* The Hague, Netherlands: Martinus Nijhoff.

Heidegger, M. (1962). *Being and time.* New York: Harper & Row.

Heidegger, M. (Ed.). (1975). The anaximander fragment. *Early Greek Thinking.* New York: Harper & Row.

Heidegger, M. (Ed.). (1975). The nature of language. *On The Way to Language.* New York: Harper & Row.

Heidegger, M. (1975). *Poetry, language and thought.* New York: Harper & Row.

Hora, T. (1961). Transcendence and healing. *Journal of Existential Psychiatry, 1,* 501.

Husserl, E. (1970). *The crisis of European sciences and transcendental phenomenology.* Evanston, IL: Northwestern University Press.

Husserl, E. (1977). *Phenomenological psychology.* The Hague, Netherlands: Martinus Nijhoff.

Ihde, D. (1983). *Existential Technics.* Albany, NY: State University of New York Press.

Ihde, D., & Zaney, R. (Eds.). (1977). *Interdisciplinary phenomenology.* The Hague, Netherlands: Martinus Nijhoff.

Johnson, R. E. (1975). *In quest of a new psychology.* New York: Human Sciences Press.

Koch, S. (1964). Psychology and emerging concepts of science as unitary. In T. Wann (Ed.), *Behaviorism and Phenomenology: Contrasting Basis for Modern Psychology.* Chicago: University of Chicago Press.

Kohler, W. (1947). *Gestalt psychology: An introduction to new concepts in psychology.* New York: Liveright.

Levin, D. (1983). The poetic function in phenomenological discourse. In W. McBride & C. Schrag (Eds.), *Phenomenology in a Pluralistic Context.* Albany, NY: State University of New York Press.

Lewin, K. (1935). *A dynamic theory of personality.* New York: McGraw-Hill.

Marton, F. (1981). Phenomenography—Describing conceptions of the world around us. *Instructional Science, 10,* 177–200.

Maslow, A. H. (1968). *Toward a psychology of being* (2nd ed.). Princeton, NJ: Van Nostrand.

McBride, W. L., & Schrag, C. O. (Eds.). (1983). *Phenomenology in a pluralistic context.* Albany, NY: State University of New York Press.

Merleau-Ponty, M. (1962). *Phenomenology of perception.* London: Routledge & Kegan.

Merleau-Ponty, M. (1964). *The primacy of perception.* Evanston, IL: Northwestern University Press.

Mohanty, J. N. (1983). The destiny of transcendental philosophy. In W.L. McBride & C.O. Schrag (Eds.), *Phenomenology in a Pluralistic Context.* Albany, NY: State University of New York Press.

Munhall, P. L. (1982). Nursing philosophy and nursing research: In apposition or opposition? *Nursing Research, 31,* 176, 177, 181.

Oiler, C. (1982). The phenomenological approach in nursing research. *Nursing Research, 31,* 178–181.

Omery, A. (1982). Phenomenology: A method for nursing research. *Advances in Nursing Science, 5*(2), 49–63.

Pivcevic, E. (Ed.). (1975). *Phenomenology and philosophical understanding.* London: Cambridge University Press.

Psathas, G. (1977). Ethnomethodology as a phenomenological approach in the social sciences. In D. Ihde & R. Zaner (Eds.), *Interdisciplinary Phenomenology.* The Hague, Netherlands: Martinus-Nijhoff.

Psathas, G. (1973). *Phenomenological sociology: Issues and applications.* New York: Wiley, 1973.

Sartre, J. (1956). *Being and Nothingness.* New York: Philosophical Library.

Spiegelberg, H. (1970). On some human uses of phenomenology. In F. J. Smith (Ed.), *Phenomenology in Perspective.* The Hague, Netherlands: Martinus Nijhoff.

Spiegelberg, H. (1965). *The Phenomenological Movement* (vol. 2). The Hague, Netherlands: Martinus Nijhoff.

Straus, E. (1966). *Phenomenological Psychology.* New York: Basic Books.

Tillich, P. (1952). *The courage to be.* New Haven, CT: Yale University Press.

Tolstoy, L. (1968). *The wisdom of Tolstoy.* New York: Philosophical Library. (Translated by Huntington Smith as an abridgement of Tolstoy, L. [1889]. *My Religion.* London: Walter Scott.)

Valle, R. S., & King, M. (Eds.). (1978). *Existential phenomenological alternatives for psychology.* New York: Oxford University Press.

Van Kaam, A. (1966). *Existential foundations of psychology* (vol. 3). Pittsburgh, PA: Duquesne University Press.

Van Kaam, A. (1959). Phenomenological analysis: Exemplified by a study of the experience of being really understood. *Individual Psychology, 15,* 66–72.

Vaught, C. G. (1983). *The quest for wholeness.* Albany, NY: State University of New York Press.

Watson, J. (1979). *Nursing: The philosophy and science of caring.* Boston: Little, Brown.

Watson, J. (1981). Professional identity crisis—Is nursing finally growing up? *American Journal of Nursing, 2,* 1488–1490.

Watson, J. (1976). Supporting materials for and introduction to the new undergraduate curriculum. Unpublished. University of Colorado School of Nursing.

Yalom, J. D. (1975). *The theory and practice of group psychotherapy* (2nd ed.). New York: Basic Books.

Zaner, R. (1975). On the sense of method in phenomenology. In E. Pivcevic (Ed.), *Phenomenology and Philosophical Understanding.* London: Cambridge University Press.

Zubek, J. P. (Ed.). (1969). *Sensory deprivation.* New York: Appleton-Century-Crofts.

CHAPTER 11

Transcendental or Depth Phenomenology and Poetic Results—An Exemplar

One further development of empirical phenomenology is the method referred to as transcendental or depth phenomenology.* This section elaborates on the extension of empirical phenomenology to the notion of transcendental–poetic expression of phenomenology. The section concludes with excerpts of transcendental poetry that capture the same experience as the empirical approach but present it in very different language.

Phenomenology takes the position that phenomenology is not just a descriptive methodology but a poetic formulation of language that attempts to interpret experiential evidence and dynamics (Levin, 1983a). The notion of transcendental phenomenology has been described as "a powerful guardian of the dream we name, echoing an earlier renaissance, the dream of humanism" (Levin, 1983b, p. 217).

The humanism in phenomenology consists of the capacity of this experiential methodology to be a method of self-awareness and self-understanding that contributes "not only to our satisfaction but can guide us toward a well-being that really fulfills our human nature" (Levin, 1983b, p. 217). Transcendental phenomenology is concerned with the very depth of experience and an openness to our nature, our potential for being. Thus, in being true to depth, openness, and humanism, transcendental phenomenology requires an experiential depth and is indeed transcendental (of pure facts and descriptions) insofar as it "cherishes the process of deepening and opening and nurtures with methodological guidance a continuing movement of self-transcendence" (Levin, 1983c, p. 218).

Husserl realized that the transcendental method gives access to a hidden or deep realm of experience that functions according to inwrought principles of its own order, without being obliged to rectify it as an objective-factual thought, but rather to consider the deeply rich experiential process as a form of transcendence from the experience itself (Levin, 1983c,d).

---

*This section is drawn from the work of David Levin (1983).

The transcendental notion in this sense acknowledges "the inexhaustible depth and openness of the implicit treasury of human experiences" (Levin, 1983d, p. 218). According to Merleau-Ponty, the transcendental method is not a means of establishing an autonomous transcendental subjectivity, but rather a gesture that initiates "the perpetual beginning of reflection, at the point where the individual life begins to reflect on itself" (Merlau-Ponty, 1962, p. 62).

In this sense then, transcendental or depth phenomenology is very closely aligned with art and science in that it is the act of bringing truth of an experience into being. As such, transcendental phenomenology is an almost perfect methodological match for studying and developing nursing as a human science and art, and researching the human care process described as transpersonal caring.

In numerous instances in this work I have attempted to make a case for why and how the traditional quantitative methods were inconsistent with nursing subject matter and premises related to nursing being a human science and art. In this last section, I am taking that position a step further. Based on my philosophy and my view of science, humans, and nursing, it is also necessary to abandon the original Husserlian vision of phenomenology being a *rigorous phenomenological science* and the paradigm that the method is *pure description*. According to Merleau-Ponty (1962), Levin (1983), and others, to envision phenomenology as pure description places it within the outdated paradigm of rationalism and logical positivism rather than within an approach that is true to the vital and creative dimension of depth experience; indeed, an approach that achieves a "poetic" effect in that the articulations of the experience, as felt and lived, transcend the facts and pure description of the experiences. As such, transcendental phenomenology allows for some poetic ambiguity, some sensuous resonance, characteristic of an experiential approach to study, but a conception of description that helps us to focus on our experience and bring it into expression.

The methodological analysis and procedure adopted by Giorgi (1975), Alexandersson (1981), and Marton (1981), presented in the previous section, as innovative and nontraditional as they may seem, are examples of the more traditional orthodox phenomenological approach to experience. However, Merleau-Ponty, Levin, and others allow for the phenomenologist researcher to go beyond the surface phenomenology and relate the description to the depth and openness of experience; this method allows reflection on the experience, the process of emergent meaning, insight, and the actual expression of the experience take into account the dynamic movement involved in the process of reflecting and using language. The result is or can be poetic. The result unites science with art.

As the researcher allows for the level of depth or transcendence of the description of the experience to contact another dimension of one's being, which taps depth and openness, there is potential for being oneself and being true to oneself. As we allow this to occur, however, we find ourselves in touch with much more than the fact, the pure description, and in touch with much more of our being than we can know in a cognitive, intellectual way.

Whenever such transcendence occurs the descriptions of the phenomeno-logical experience never truly fit the experience; there remains an elusiveness and an ambiguity in the meanings. However, the transcendent data as presented have the potential to allow the researcher to be true to his or her self and acknowledge the openness of the process. To be true to one's self and the depth of humanism in which phenomenology is embedded, one must acknowledge the openness of the process and also stay with it in "truthful harmony, because openness to our being is the center, the heart of our essential nature" (Levin, 1983e).

To further quote Levin (1983e) "if there be any truth, then, in the transcen-dental method (of phenomenology), it must be that the transcendental is not just a method for understanding the facticity of experience; but that it is also a way of enjoying, or appreciating the intrinsically creative and open nature of experiences, because appreciation of this nature is a necessary condition for true and authentic existential knowledge."

Therefore, if phenomenology is to be true to the human science and art of nursing and the human care process, it must penetrate beneath the surface of familiar, habitually organized, and standardized experience. What is at issue is pre-senting the phenomenological experience; in the use of language, as such, the lan-guage must have a transcendental and no longer a mundane relationship to our experience. The process of transcendental phenomenology commits us to a lan-guage that encourages existential authenticity. Moreover, authentic speech that is true to experience, and also true to our deepest experience of expression, is languaging that touches and opens up the transformative process (Levin, 1983e).

According to Levin, "authentic languaging, trascendentally gets involved in the potential for growth implied in our reflection-upon-experience." This dif-ference is not so much a question of their different contexts of meaning as it is a question of their way of relating to the experiential process. The transcen-dental reduction does not change the meaning of our words; rather, it changes how our words relate to the experience (Levin, 1983e). For example, an Abo-riginal does not own land, the land owns him. It's an entirely different rela-tionship, one to another. Therefore, in acknowledging the transcendental nature of both the human experience of phenomenology as well as the nature of its expression, it is necessary to acknowledge that the way in which experience is expressed is at least as important as the content, the facts, and the pure description of the experience.

We cannot convey the need for compassion, complexity, or for cultivating feeling and sensibility in words that are bereft of warmth, kindness, and good feeling (Levin, 1983f).

For phenomenology to be true to humanism of experience, the language used to describe the experience must penetrate beneath the factual surface of everyday experience and allow us to see anew, to address a powerful truth that moves us to realize our deepest tendencies and existential meaningfulness (Levin, 1983e) (to allow for release of feelings one has been longing and wishing to express).

In the ideas of Heidegger (1975a) the result is poetizing (Dichtung), which is the true vocation of the experiential phenomenologist. According to Levin again, poetizing, in this instance, is necessary in that transcendental depth phenomenology, if focused and reflective of depth human experiences, cannot be other than poetic (Levin, 1983f). This occurs first by expressing and conveying—embodying—the beautifully good feeling that spontaneously arises with the saying of that which is true to experience, and second, by virtue of this truth (being-in-truth), disclosing a more open space. Poetizing addresses and lays claim to our potential for being, and, like a metaphor, it carries us forward.

To continue in Levin's words (Levin, 1983g, p. 229):

> Any experiential articulation that (1) is rooted in a truly felt experience, (2) emerges from that experience in a felt movement of self-expression, and (3) maintains its contact with the original, spontaneous thrust of experience, even in the phase of completed expression, will at least tend to be (tend to sound) poetic.

He goes on to conclude that, "in phenomenological discourse, therefore, the deepest transcendental truth of an existentially authentic languaging of experience will be articulated with the sensuous resonance, the emotional spaciousness, and the elemental openness of the poetic word."

Heidegger (1971) referred to the importance of actually undergoing an experience with language and letting our experiences speak for themselves. He indicated we should let ourselves be transformed by our participation in the process (Heidegger (1975b). Moreover, poetic expression has the power to touch and move us, to open and transport us. Thus, the poetic quality is related to the experiential meaning and, indeed, deepens the meaning, the felt senses, so that there is increased openness to describe and preserve the truth and depth of the experience.

Indeed, when a phenomenologist is true to the depths of the moving human experience, he or she almost naturally poetizes. Levin suggests that poetizing descriptions of transcendental phenomenology serves as visualizations and imaginative projections. As such, the power of imagination through poetizing actually brings us nearer to a way of being (we are already living) and moves us deeper into that open transcendental realm of experience.

If we are to consider this deep level of phenomenology, that is beyond pure descriptions, and allow for the transcendental experience as both felt and expressed through poetic language, then we have to give up the correspondence theory of truth and adapt the aletheia theory of truth that is associated with discovery of the unknown or unconcealment (Marton, 1981). We also have to abandon the notion of a "descriptive" as well as "factual," "quantitative" truth that simply corresponds to facts and figures. The human science and art of nursing and human care, which are indeed transpersonal, must incorporate feeling, depth of experience, and transcendental processes that result in poetic expression, which move us toward authentic experiential expression and help us maintain openness with our humanism and our potential for growth. Finally, transcendental phenomenology also reminds us that, as nurses, in either practice or research efforts, we are first of all human beings, capable of transcending the moment, capable of engaging in a truly felt experience, emerging from that experience with a desire for self-expression while still being capable of maintaining contact with the original, spontaneous thrust of the experience.

Example of Transcendental Phenomenology and Poetic Expression

As a way of capturing transcendental phenomenology, I am concluding with excerpts of original poetry written immediately after my phenomenological research experience with an Aboriginal tribe in Western Australia.

Incidentally, the writing of the poetry was in itself a transcendent experience for me. As I left the Aboriginal mission and the other friends in Kalgoorlie, Western Australia, I was faced with an overnight train ride back to civilization in Perth, the coastal city. During the train ride I had an overwhelming desire to express my feelings and capture the gestalt of my experience and also to capture the gestalt of the Aborigines' loss-caring experiences. In reflecting back on my field notes, the data, and the entire experience, the poetic expression formulated on the overnight train ride captures the truth of the experience and the meaning of the human phenomena better than any factual data described without any feeling of personal involvement. The transcendental description was rooted in a truly felt experience that indeed transcended the here and now and resulted in a much more comprehensive expression of the deeply human experiential process.

Dreamtime and Sharing the Tears with Wongi Tribe of Cundeelee

Jean Watson, Western Australia, May 1982

An arch of eyebrows
that represents the bush
of the Bush Country he comes from,
has left and is now longing to return to.
With his sugar bag he is preparing
to return home
      to his people
before the end and after
      the reburial.
The "time out" of grief is
approaching two years or longer.
When he's ready he'll let
      his people know.
His dark skin, so dark
around his eyes
I have to look two or three times
to catch the shine of the brown eyes
      that know all,
        see all, yet are.
He speaks about visions, the Milky Way,
the black hole,
they told him in Dreamtime.

His people have known
      for thousands of years.
The end will come when
the black hole is in the
Milky Way and the Emu
      in the stars
makes a drumming noise.
The heavens will open at
      the black hole.
You can see the religious awakening
happening all over the world.

There's that side of Bill
and then there's the power of the
      Spirit
I felt in the dark
of Cundeelee Camp.
We floundered and wondered

how it would be to talk—
      whether he would "see" and
I could be real with him.

And we spoke
      and left it—
Spoke and
      left it.
I wandered to be alone in the
      dark of Cundeelee.
The steps outside
the sister's compound.
The ashes of the coals
The fire of Mangrove Root
Chanting children
Singing of God
"If you're happy and you know it
clap your hands."
He stepped up to me
I felt it.
      The warm flow of
his acceptance
his approval
his readiness
      to be with me.
It came from my throat
      and chest
and moved to him
      with warmth
and enclosed me.
The words didn't matter.
      I couldn't hear.
But we both knew it was
      okay.
But others kept coming, talking
      noises and words.
Time, Patience
The group gathering—
      the Elders
      red head bands
The eldest with cowboy hat.

The women and children
      naked and dressed.

The dingoes all gathered
        to fill the soul
with singing, and clapping
and telling their woes.
The sins, the drinking, the
        tearing their souls.
The visions, the hurts,
        the finding the Lord.
The arrows that pointed
        from the clouds above
and led them to Christ,
        the Son, the Lord,
and now they had come
        to spread the Word.

All questioning and listening
and singing their songs.
Bill came up and told me
so specially so "I want you
        to have some of my kangaroo tail."
I floundered, but nodded
I was pleased to accept, not
knowing what ritual presented
        itself.

After watching Bill peel it
        of skin and fur, I reckoned
        I ate it, instead of observe.
So, little by little with proper
        bites,
I daintily abided his
        appetite.
Gourmet?, not really—but
        surely not bad.
To taste a little oily
        kangaroo tail.
But then came the photos
to catch it all live—cause
no one would believe me
back in American eyes.

Struggling and trying to
        find my way.
Do I look out to the

people
or hide in their ways?
Bill taught me that hiding the eyes
may be better for them
to capture the wholeness
without rude chagrin.
And then came the Elders.
The men of the tribe who
asked for Bill's counsel
to help them decide what
someone from Boulder could
possibly do with people as
remote as
Aborigines from Cundeelee.

He tried to express
with his best Wongi tongue
"That lady's a Sister,
a nurse;
a bloke if you will
who seeketh the wisdom
of you and me,
The feelings of people from Cundeelee."

The caring and loss concepts
of Aboriginal disgrace
so beautifully spelt, but so
ineptly expressed.
Bill had the words, the signs and
the grace
to explain it all kindly
to the full men without haste.
He used words of the
Wongi
that left me behind
but carried the men to
Dreamtime Beyond.
His white head of wisdom,
he knew beyond all—
the right way to cross over
the lands that bind—
the hearts that twine
when the worlds unfold.
I found myself stumbling

when they knew it all.
They said it like this.
It's a world behind in Dreamtime,
it's finished
    we're free
after proper "time out" to
    clear the head—
of headaches, the memories,
the sorrow and grief.
The Wongi for Caring
    means "sharing the tears"
But after the comfort,
which includes an embrace,
that only then tells us
    You care for our race.

We also want help
    to get to our nearest place
to find our relatives
to carry on the debate
And how to release
    the Community
    from the State
The State that denies them
    the "time out" they need
    to fill up their sorrow
    pour out the grief

The greed of the Country,
    the business, the mines
That won't let the people
    wail as they need
When all they ask for
    is time out to grieve.

It's so deep, so painful
They say it all hurts
They must be alone to
    properly mourn
Even if it includes
    some self abuse
That white man can't conger
    so obtuse
Cause our fields are

from Dreamtime
that penetrates years
and guides all our people
to bury their fears
to trust one another
and learn to obey
to believe in our brothers
in spite of their ways.
To wish for them goodness
even when they pray
regardless of memories
and haunting decay.

They sit and they hope
they sleep in the night
beyond all comprehension
of white man's likes.

They watch in the heavens
for the Milky Way paths
Emu noises and black holes
That quake.
The earth, The water, The birds
and The fowl,
The animals and trees
and certainly the tail of
The lowliest Kangaroo
that shivers and quails.
When all men are gone
according to scale.
We knew it all through hundreds
of stories. Dreamtime continues to wail.
The grief you say is only one tale

The forefather's Dreamtimes
are mighty and powerful
and all we entail.
The earth is our partner
our part of this life
It's sacred to feel
and sinful to fail.

The Dreamtime shows us
how never to err

When it comes to uncovering
> The rocks and the soil,
Because of the death and
> destruction that's left
> in the trail.
Instead of objects and gemstones
> and people with dreams
But only death and destruction
> Youla—I mean
Even the name change
> to Yolaria
> Can't change the time
> That's played for Mankind
> once the notes are produced.

So leave it alone, don't tamper
> with fate
The Uranium's a hate of
> the whole human race
Except the miners and sharers
> of great
The Dreamers of Visions
for money and fame;
> for rights and lights and
> claims are at stake.

But listen to wisdom to time
> and my stories of late
That have been told by the
> Dreamtime and hold us
> awake
If only we hear The children
> and chants in the night
The stars in the heavens
> That show us what's right
The soul's reawakening will
> come in the night
If you listen to Dreamtime
> before all goes quiet.

Wongi reminders will haunt
> after all
When Cundeelee mission
> has nowhere to fall.

REFERENCES

Alexandersson, C. (1981). Amedeo Giorgi's empirical phenomenology (publication no. 3). Swedish Council for Research in Humanities and Social Sciences, Department of Education, University of Goteborg, Goteborg, Sweden, *3*, 1–35.

Giorgi, A. (1975). An application of phenomenological method in psycholody. In A. Giorgi, C. Fisher, & E. Murray (Eds), *Duquesne studies in phenomenological psychology*, (vol. 2, pp. 82–84). Pittsburgh, PA: Dusquesne University Press.

Heidegger, M. (Ed.). (1971).The nature of language. *On the way to language* (p. 98). New York, NY: Harper & Row.

Heidegger, M. (1975a). *Poetry, language and thought* (p. 155). New York: Harper & Row.

Heidegger, M. (Ed.). (1975b). The anaximander fragment. *Early Greek thinking* (p. 155). New York: Harper & Row.

Levin, D. (1983a). The poetic function in phenomenological discourse. In W. McBride and C. Schrag (Eds.), *Phenomenology in a pluralistic context* (pp. 216–234). Albany, NY: State University of New York Press.

Levin, D. (1983b). The poetic function in phenomenological discourse. In W. McBride and C. Schrag (Eds.), *Phenomenology in a pluralistic context* (p. 217). Albany, NY: State University of New York Press.

Levin, D. (1983c). The poetic function in phenomenological discourse. In W. McBride and C. Schrag (Eds.), *Phenomenology in a pluralistic context* (p. 218). Albany, NY: State University of New York Press.

Levin, D. (1983d). The poetic function in phenomenological discourse. In W. McBride and C. Schrag (Eds.), *Phenomenology in a pluralistic context* (pp. 218–219). Albany, NY: State University of New York Press.

Levin, D. (1983e). The poetic function in phenomenological discourse. In W. McBride and C. Schrag (Eds.), *Phenomenology in a pluralistic context* (p. 221). Albany, NY: State University of New York Press.

Levin, D. (1983f). The poetic function in phenomenological discourse. In W. McBride and C. Schrag (Eds), *Phenomenology in a pluralistic context* (p. 228). Albany, NY: State University of New York Press.

Levin, D. (1983g). The poetic function in phenomenological discourse. In W. McBride and C. Schrag (Eds.), *Phenomenology in a pluralistic context* (p. 229). Albany, NY: State University of New York Press.

Marton, E. (1981). Phenomenology—Describing conceptions of the world around us. *Instructional Science, 10*, 177–200.

Merleau-Ponty, M. (1962). *Phenomenology of perception*. London, England: Routledge & Kegan.

Index

A
Adaptation, concept of, 9f, 10
Aletheia theory of truth, 107
Alexandersson, C., 96, 97, 104
Art
    Nightingale's view on, 18–19
    transcendental phenomenology and, 104
Authenticity
    of human experience, 94–95, 98–99, 105
    individuality and, 81
    in listening, 79
    ontology and, 93–94

B
Baldwin, B., 21
Bateson, Mary Catherine, 83
Benner, P., 12, 18
Biocidic caring, 45, 46
Biogenic caring, 45–46
Biopassive caring, 45, 46
Biostatic caring, 45, 46
Boykin, A., 12, 18
Bronowski, J., 1

C
Caring/human caring
    bicidic-biogenic continuum, 45
    conditions for, 42
    cross-cultural data on, 44–45
    definition of, 38
    demonstration/practice of, 43–44
    elements in, 38
    human-to-human process of, 19, 75
    moral commitment to, 41, 42
    as moral ideal of nursing, 38, 41, 65, 75
    noncaring and, 44–46
    nonmedical processes of, 20
    in nursing, 35, 45 (*See also* Human caring
        science nursing paradigm)
    preservation/advancement of, 43
    processes in, 44
    in scientific models, 7
    temporal/spatial aspect of, 45
    threats to, 43
    transpersonal (*See* Transpersonal caring)
    as universal, 63
    values of (*See* Caring values)
    Watson's carative factors/processes, 46, 47t
Caring-healing modalities, in theory of
    human care, 89–90
Caring values
    actions and, 41–42
    consciousness and, 41–42
    in nursing, assumptions of, 42–44
    in theory of human care, 88–89
    Watson's value system of, 46, 47t
Chinn, P., 21, 93
Community health nursing, 37
Concepts, 4–10. *See also specific concepts*
    balanced view of, 5
    continua (*See* Concrete-abstract
        continuum; Static-dynamic
        continuum)
    in non-nursing disciplines, 7
    starting point for, 5–7
Concrete-abstract continuum
    description of, 4–5, 4f, 6f
    Rogers' concept of energy field and,
        9–10, 9f
    Roy's adaptation concept and, 9f, 10
    theory development phases and, 8–9
    theory of human care and, 7–8, 8f
Congruence-incongruence continuum, 68–69
Consciousness
    caring values and, 41–42
    continuity over time, 67
    "cosmic," 50
    higher sense of, 58
    soul and, 62
    in theory of human care, 87–88
    toward unitary world view (*See* World
        view, unitary)
Cook, T., 26
Correspondence theory of truth, 107

D
Davis, A., 21
de Chardin, T., 42, 43, 62, 63, 67, 88
Depth phenomenology. *See* Transcendental
    depth phenomenology
Discourse, phenomenological, 106
Dock, L., 50